AF725008

Field Surgery of Cattle, Part II

Guest Editor

DAVID E. ANDERSON, DVM, MS
MATT D. MIESNER, DVM, MS

VETERINARY CLINICS
OF NORTH AMERICA:
FOOD ANIMAL PRACTICE

www.vetfood.theclinics.com

Consulting Editor
ROBERT A. SMITH, DVM, MS

November 2008 • Volume 24 • Number 3

SAUNDERS an imprint of ELSEVIER, Inc.

W.B. SAUNDERS COMPANY
A Division of Elsevier Inc.

1600 John F. Kennedy Boulevard • Suite 1800 • Philadelphia, PA 19103-2899

http://www.vetfood.theclinics.com

VETERINARY CLINICS OF NORTH AMERICA: FOOD ANIMAL PRACTICE Volume 24, Number 3 November 2008 ISSN 0749-0720, ISBN-13: 978-1-4160-6372-8, ISBN-10: 1-4160-6372-2

Editor: John Vassallo; j.vassallo@elsevier.com

© **2008 Elsevier ■ All rights reserved.**

This journal and the individual contributions contained in it are protected under copyright by Elsevier, and the following terms and conditions apply to their use:

Photocopying
Single photocopies of single articles may be made for personal use as allowed by national copyright laws. Permission of the Publisher and payment of a fee is required for all other photocopying, including multiple or systematic copying, copying for advertising or promotional purposes, resale, and all forms of document delivery. Special rates are available for educational institutions that wish to make photocopies for non-profit educational classroom use. For information on how to seek permission visit www.elsevier.com/permissions or call: (+44) 1865 843830 (UK)/(+1) 215 239 3804 (USA).

Derivative Works
Subscribers may reproduce tables of contents or prepare lists of articles including abstracts for internal circulation within their institutions. Permission of the Publisher is required for resale or distribution outside the institution. Permission of the Publisher is required for all other derivative works, including compilations and translations (please consult www.elsevier.com/permissions).

Electronic Storage or Usage
Permission of the Publisher is required to store or use electronically any material contained in this journal, including any article or part of an article (please consult www.elsevier.com/permissions). Except as outlined above, no part of this publication may be reproduced, stored in a retrieval system or transmitted in any form or by any means, electronic, mechanical, photocopying, recording or otherwise, without prior written permission of the Publisher.

Notice
No responsibility is assumed by the Publisher for any injury and/or damage to persons or property as a matter of products liability, negligence or otherwise, or from any use or operation of any methods, products, instructions or ideas contained in the material herein. Because of rapid advances in the medical sciences, in particular, independent verification of diagnoses and drug dosages should be made.

Although all advertising material is expected to conform to ethical (medical) standards, inclusion in this publication does not constitute a guarantee or endorsement of the quality or value of such product or of the claims made of it by its manufacturer.

Veterinary Clinics of North America: Food Animal Practice (ISSN 0749-0720) is published in March, July, and November by Elsevier Inc., 360 Park Avenue South, New York, NY 10010-1710. Business and Editorial Offices: 1600 John F. Kennedy Blvd., Suite 1800, Philadelphia, PA 19103-2899. Customer Service Office: 11830 Westline Industrial Drive, St. Louis, MO 63146. Periodicals postage paid at New York, NY and additional mailing offices. Subscription prices are $163.00 per year (domestic individuals), $260.00 per year (domestic institutions), $81.00 per year (domestic students/residents), $189.00 per year (Canadian individuals), $339.00 per year (Canadian institutions), $239.00 per year (international individuals), $339.00 per year (international institutions), and $123.00 per year (international and Canadian students/residents). To receive student/resident rate, orders must be accompained by name of affiliated institution, date of term, and the *signature* of program/residency coordinator on institution letterhead. Orders will be billed at individual rate until proof of status is received. Foreign air speed delivery is included in all *Clinics* subscription prices. All prices are subject to change without notice. **POSTMASTER:** Send address changes to *Veterinary Clinics of North America*: *Food Animal Practice*, 11830 Westline Industrial Drive, St. Louis, MO 63146. Customer Service (orders, claims, online, change of address): Elsevier Periodicals Customer Service, 11830 Westline Industrial Drive, St. Louis, MO 63146. Tel: 1-800-654-2452 (U.S. and Canada). Fax: 314-523-5170. E-mail: journalscustomerservice-usa@elsevier.com (for print support); journalsonlinesupport-usa@elsevier.com (for online support).

Reprints. For copies of 100 or more, of articles in this publication, please contact the Commercial Reprints Department, Elsevier Inc., 360 Park Avenue South, New York, NY 10010-1710. Tel.: 212-633-3812; Fax: 212-462-1935; E-mail: reprints@elsevier.com.

Veterinary Clinics of North America: Food Animal Practice is covered in *Current Contents/Agriculture, Biology and Environmental Sciences, MEDLINE/PubMed (Index Medicus), and Excerpta Medica.*

Printed in the United States of America.

Contributors

GUEST EDITORS

DAVID E. ANDERSON, DVM, MS
Diplomate, American College of Veterinary Surgeons; Professor and Head of Agricultural Practices, Department of Clinical Sciences, College of Veterinary Medicine, Kansas State University, Manhattan, Kansas

MATT D. MIESNER, DVM, MS
Diplomate, American College of Veterinary Internal Medicine (Large Animal Internal Medicine); Clinical Assistant Professor of Agricultural Practices, Department of Clinical Sciences, College of Veterinary Medicine, Kansas State University, Manhattan, Kansas

AUTHORS

ERIC J. ABRAHAMSEN, DVM
Diplomate, American College of Veterinary Anesthesiologists; Ocala Equine Hospital, Ocala, Florida

ANDREW J. ALLEN, DVM
Senior Resident, Department of Veterinary Clinical Sciences, Washington State University, Pullman, Washington

DAVID E. ANDERSON, DVM, MS
Diplomate, American College of Veterinary Surgeons; Professor and Head of Agricultural Practices, Department of Clinical Sciences, College of Veterinary Medicine, Kansas State University, Manhattan, Kansas

AUBREY N. BAIRD, DVM, MS
Diplomate, American College of Veterinary Surgeons; Associate Professor and Chief of Large Animal Surgery, Department of Veterinary Clinical Sciences, School of Veterinary Medicine, Purdue University, West Lafayette, Indiana

GEORGE M. BARRINGTON, DVM, PhD
Diplomate, American College of Veterinary Internal Medicine; Assistant Professor, Department of Veterinary Clinical Sciences, Washington State University, Pullman, Washington

LIONEL J. DAWSON, BVSc, MS
Diplomate, American College of Theriogenologists; Center for Veterinary Health Sciences, Oklahoma State University, Stillwater; American Institute for Goat Research, Langston University, Langston, Oklahoma

ANDRÉ DESROCHERS, DMV, MS
Diplomate, American College of Veterinary Surgeons; Diplomate, European College of Bovine Health Management; Professor and Head, Farm Animal Medicine and Surgery, Department of Clinical Sciences, Université de Montréal, Saint-Hyacinthe, Quebec, Canada

JENNIFER M. EWOLDT, DVM, MS
Diplomate, American College of Veterinary Surgeons; Scott County Animal Hospital, Eldridge, Iowa

MEREDYTH L. JONES, DVM, MS
Diplomate, American College of Veterinary Internal Medicine; Department of Clinical Sciences, Kansas State University, Manhattan, Kansas

MIREILLE MEYLAN, Dr med vet, FVH, MS, PhD, Dr habil
Diplomate, American College of Veterinary Internal Mediicne (Large Animal Internal Medicine); Diplomate, European College of Bovine Health Management; Associate Professor, Clinic for Ruminants, Vetsuisse Faculty of the University of Berne, Berne, Switzerland

MATT D. MIESNER, DVM, MS
Diplomate, American College of Veterinary Internal Medicine (Large Animal Internal Medicine); Clinical Assistant Professor of Agricultural Practices, Department of Clinical Sciences, College of Veterinary Medicine, Kansas State University, Manhattan, Kansas

GREGOR L. MORGAN, BVSc, MS, PhD
Diplomate, American College of Theriogenologists; Associate Professor, Center for Veterinary Health Sciences, Oklahoma State University, Stillwater, Oklahoma

STEVE M. PARISH, DVM
Diplomate, American College of Veterinary Internal Medicine; Professor, Department of Veterinary Clinical Sciences, Washington State University, Pullman, Washington

KARA SCHULZ, DVM
Instructor, Agricultural Practices, Department of Clinical Sciences, College of Veterinary Medicine, Kansas State University, Manhattan, Kansas

GUY ST. JEAN, DMV, MS
Diplomate, American College of Veterinary Surgeons; Associate Dean for Academic Affairs, Ross University School of Veterinary Medicine, Basseterre, Saint Kitts, West Indies

Contents

Veterinary Clinics of North America: Food Animal Practice

FORTHCOMING ISSUES

March 2009

Bovine Neonatology

Geof Smith, DVM, PhD, *Guest Editor*

July 2009

Camelids

David E. Anderson, DVM, MS and
Claire E. Whitehead, BVM&S, MS, MRCVS,
Guest Editors

November 2009

Food Animal Ultrasound

Sébastien Buczinski, Dr Vét,
Guest Editor

RECENT ISSUES

July 2008

Field Surgery of Cattle, Part I

David E. Anderson, DVM, MS and
Matt D. Miesner, DVM, MS, *Guest Editors*

March 2008

Dairy Heifer Management

Sandra Godden, DVM, DVSc and
Sheila M. McGuirk, DVM, PhD,
Guest Editors

November 2007

Ruminant Diagnostic Medicine

Robert J. Callan, DVM, MS, PhD,
Guest Editor

RELATED INTEREST

Veterinary Clinics of North America: Equine Practice April 2007 (Vol. 23, No. 1)
Trauma and Emergency Care
Eileen K. Sullivan, DVM, MS, *Guest Editor*

THE CLINICS ARE NOW AVAILABLE ONLINE!

Access your subscription at:
www.theclinics.com

Preface

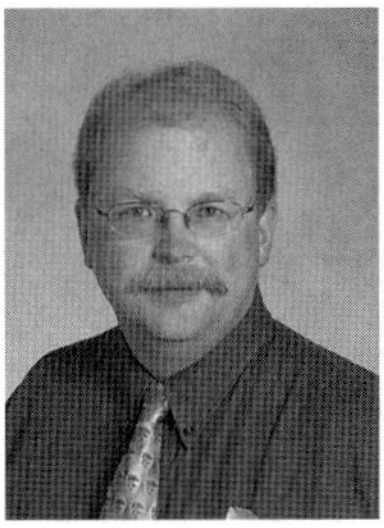
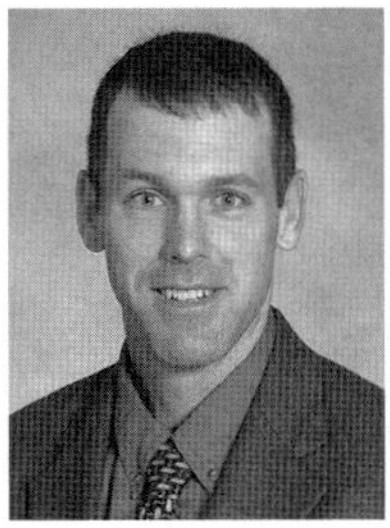

David E. Anderson, DVM, MS Matt D. Miesner, DVM, MS
Guest Editors

This text completes the two-part series on "Field Surgery of Cattle" that began with the July 2008 issue. This issue continues to build upon information and techniques in soft tissue surgery and includes considerably more information regarding orthopedics. Advances in surgical materials, anesthetic drugs, and physiologic application make difficult surgical procedures more approachable in bovine patients in the field.

Tremendous advances have taken place in food animal practice, especially in the area of production medicine. Surgery on food animals still is performed routinely and is performed primarily in field settings. The ability to diagnose and manage surgical problems is one basis for gaining the trust and confidence of the client. Economic and other constraints often prevent cattle from being referred to surgical centers for specialized care. Again, advanced topics are included, but they are written in light of on-farm capabilities.

Animal pain and welfare are serious issues. To that end, we include detailed articles on nerve blocks, chemical restraint, and anesthesia to facilitate surgical procedures in the most humane manner possible. The authors endorse alleviation of pain whenever possible, and the contents of these issues should aid in that goal.

David E. Anderson, DVM, MS
Matt D. Miesner, DVM, MS
Department of Clinical Sciences
College of Veterinary Medicine
Kansas State University
1800 Denison Avenue
Manhattan, KS 66506, USA

E-mail addresses:
danderso@vet.ksu.edu (D.E. Anderson)
mmiesner@vet.k-state.edu (M.D. Miesner)

Vet Clin Food Anim 24 (2008) xi
doi:10.1016/j.cvfa.2008.07.007 vetfood.theclinics.com
0749-0720/08/$ – see front matter © 2008 Elsevier Inc. All rights reserved.

Ruminant Field Anesthesia

Eric J. Abrahamsen, DVM

KEYWORDS

- Ketamine stun • Xylazine-ketamine • BKX • Double drip
- Ruminant triple drip • Ket-val

Ruminants can be safely anesthetized in a field setting. The higher level of analgesia provided by anesthesia eliminates the need for local anesthetic blockade, which can prove useful when a procedure is expected to produce a substantial level of pain or local anesthetic blockade is not feasible. Certain aspects of anesthesia place the patient at greater risk than chemical restraint techniques. Knowledge and vigilance reduce the additional risks associated with anesthesia.

PREANESTHETIC CONSIDERATIONS

Physical Examination

A brief physical examination should be performed, including an overall assessment of the patient's health status, auscultation of the cardiopulmonary systems, and evaluation of locomotor function. This examination helps determine if the patient is a suitable candidate for field anesthesia and may reduce liability should anesthetic complications occur.

Site Selection

A flat, even surface that provides good footing should be selected. The surface should be soft to help protect against injury during induction and recovery. The site selected should be free of hazards in all directions. Large ruminants are more difficult to physically control and require a somewhat larger safety zone. Ruminants tend to be patient during recovery from anesthesia. They typically do not attempt to stand until they are awake and functional. Good footing is the primary requirement for achieving a good recovery. An open grassy area is generally ideal. A stall deeply bedded with shavings can be used, but the confined space increases risk for personnel involved and may interfere with the procedure. Proximity to water, electricity, and a vehicle (containing emergency supplies) are also factors to consider when selecting a site. A calm environment reduces patient anxiety and is always desirable.

Ocala Equine Hospital, 10855 N.W. U.S Highway 27, Ocala, FL 34482, USA
E-mail address: abrahamsen@earthlink.net

Vet Clin Food Anim 24 (2008) 429–441
doi:10.1016/j.cvfa.2008.07.001
vetfood.theclinics.com
0749-0720/08/$ – see front matter © 2008 Published by Elsevier Inc.

Intravenous Catheters Are Expensive and Time Consuming—Are They Really Necessary?

A catheter should be placed before anesthetizing ruminant patients. The jugular vein is the most commonly used site for intravenous catheter placement. The thicker skin of ruminants makes catheter placement more difficult and accidental placement in the carotid artery has occurred. A 14-gauge 5.5-in catheter is used in most ruminant patients. An 18-gauge 2-in catheter is sufficient for lambs and kids. The catheter should be secured to the neck with suture or bandage. The catheter should always be checked before anesthetic induction to ensure it is still functional. The veins on the external surface of the ear have been used as an alternative site for venous access in ruminant patients. An 18- or 20-gauge catheter should be used and secured with a combination of super glue and tape. These smaller catheters do not provide the flow rate of the 14-gauge catheter, but work well otherwise.

Endotracheal Intubation

Ruminants continue to produce a significant amount of saliva while anesthetized. The field anesthesia techniques covered in this article tend to leave a degree of laryngeal and eye reflexes in place, but they should not be counted on to protect the airway. Ruminants anesthetized in a field setting should be positioned so that saliva runs out of the mouth rather than pooling back near the larynx. For patients in lateral recumbency this can be accomplished simply by placing a pad under the head-neck junction so that the opening of the mouth is below the level of the larynx.

Protecting the airway becomes much more challenging when the patient is placed in dorsal recumbency. Smaller ruminants placed in dorsal recumbency are generally under the influence of a potent chemical restraint technique or anesthetized. The body of these patients should be sufficiently elevated using foam pads or some other method with the head resting on the floor or surgery table surface. It is important that the head be supported rather than hanging in space to prevent excessive tension on neck structures. The head and neck are rotated to place the opening of the mouth below the larynx to facilitate saliva egress. The short thick neck of many cattle breeds can make proper orientation difficult to achieve. When the head cannot be positioned to facilitate saliva egress or the procedure is expected to produce a significant amount of blood or other material that could enter the airway the patient should be intubated. Larger ruminant patients are difficult to move, let alone lift, while anesthetized, and proper dorsal positioning is difficult to obtain in the field setting.

Many practitioners carry a selection of smaller endotracheal tubes and an Ambu bag for resuscitating newborn patients. The silicone endotracheal tubes (Bivona Aire-Cuf standard silicone endotracheal tubes with Murphy eye and connector, Smiths Medical) used in larger ruminants are expensive. Practitioners planning to anesthetize larger ruminant patients in dorsal recumbency should add a small selection of larger endotracheal tubes to the equipment in their vehicle. A compromise might be to add 12-, 16-, and 22-mm endotracheal tubes, which provide an adequate airway for a wide range of patient size. Patients weighing more than 680 kg experience increased work of breathing with a 22-mm endotracheal tube. Patients should be extubated with cuff inflated in sternal recumbency to reduce risk for aspiration.

A brief period of apnea immediately following anesthetic induction with thiopental is fairly common. The central nervous system (CNS) depression produced by the thiopental bolus elevates the respiratory set point (the $Paco_2$ level that initiates ventilation). The $Paco_2$ increases during the period of apnea, eventually reaching the new set point, and spontaneous ventilation resumes. Anesthetic induction with ketamine does not significantly alter the respiratory set point value and postinduction apnea is uncommon. Ketamine does affect the respiratory center. Irregular (apneustic) breathing is fairly common immediately following anesthetic induction with ketamine or Telazol in equine patients, although it is less common in ruminants. Apneustic breathing does not generally last long and is of little consequence in normal healthy patients unless uptake of inhalation anesthetics is involved. A 160 L/min demand valve (JDM-5041, JD Medical, Phoenix, Arizona) and portable oxygen supply (tank and pressure regulator) are required to treat prolonged apnea. There is no substitute for this equipment on the rare occasions it might be required, but justification of the expense and space required varies from practice to practice. This equipment should be standard in all large animal clinics in which anesthesia is regularly performed.

Oxygen Delivery and Muscle and Nerve Protection

Oxygen supplementation is not generally required during short-term field anesthesia in ruminants. Oxygen delivery and muscle and nerve protection are covered in greater detail in Ref. [1].

Fasting Before Anesthesia

Functioning ruminants should be fasted before anesthesia. Fasting reduces the volume of rumen contents, which reduces pressure on the diaphragm and the incidence of regurgitation. Ruminants properly fasted are less likely to bloat during recumbency and anesthesia. Withholding food and water for 24 hours before surgery has been traditionally recommended. Experience with nonfasted emergency cases has shown proper technique to be the most important factor in reducing the risk for regurgitation during induction and intubation. Attempting to intubate a patient with some degree of gag reflex present is more likely to result in regurgitation. Proper induction technique eliminates the gag reflex. Keeping the patient in sternal recumbency with the head elevated reduces the risk for passive regurgitation during intubation. Withholding food for 12 to 18 hours (access to water is permitted) has proved effective in minimizing problems during intubation and anesthesia while not producing the adverse effects on rumen motility and acid–base status associated with longer periods of fasting. Some abdominal procedures benefit from a greater reduction of rumen volume and a longer period of fasting is required in these cases.

Young animals have minimal energy stores. The risk for hypoglycemia in these patients increases with the duration of anesthesia. Nursing ruminants are typically anesthetized without fasting to reduce the risk for hypoglycemia. Ruminants less than 2 months of age should be supplemented with dextrose during anesthesia. Adding 1.25% to 2.5% dextrose to the intravenous (IV) electrolyte solution (10 mL/kg/h) is generally sufficient to ensure blood glucose levels are adequately maintained in these patients. Generally by 2 months of age most healthy ruminant patients no longer require dextrose supplementation during shorter anesthetic procedures. Adding 1.25% dextrose to the IV fluids is cheap insurance against hypoglycemia in ruminant patients 2 to 4 months of age when a long period of anesthesia is anticipated. Elevated body temperature increases metabolism and increases the risk for hypoglycemia in younger patients. Patients up to 4 months of age should be supplemented with dextrose when body temperature is significantly elevated.

Unless testing is performed during anesthesia, hypoglycemia is typically not recognized until the recovery period. Hypoglycemia produces a stuporous state and patients typically stall partway through the recovery process. Administration of dextrose has resulted in full recovery with no apparent adverse effects when this has occurred. Prevention is preferred to treatment. Protracted struggling during physical restraint of unruly young patients can produce substantial elevation of body temperature. Unruly patients should be sedated rather than battled.

Eye Protection

When ruminants are placed in lateral recumbency care should be taken to ensure the lids of the down eye are closed. A towel or thin pad can be placed under the down eye to provide further protection. Ophthalmic ointment (bland or antibiotic) should be placed in the eyes to protect them during anesthesia. If the down eye ends up bathed in saliva or regurgitation it should be rinsed out during recovery.

DRUGS USED IN RUMINANT FIELD ANESTHESIA

α_2-Adrenergic Agonists

Xylazine is the most frequently used drug for sedation in large animals. Ruminants are 10 times more sensitive to xylazine than horses, whereas detomidine is dosed similarly in both species. Ruminants tend to lie down when dosed aggressively with α_2-adrenergic agonists, whereas horses exhibit increasing levels of ataxia.

The initial demeanor of the patient greatly influences the sedation produced by a given dose of an α_2-adrenergic agonist. The sedative effect of α_2-adrenergic agonists can be overridden by elevated sympathetic tone, resulting in two characteristic features of α_2-adrenergic agonist sedation. The sedative effect produced by lower doses of α_2-adrenergic agonists is not as stable. Calm, quiet patients require smaller doses, whereas anxious or unruly patients require larger doses. This requirement sounds simple, but selecting the incorrect dose may result in working on your knees or getting kicked in them. The ideal dose can be difficult to predict, especially when recumbency is not desired. Experience makes the necessary adjustments easier, but even seasoned practitioners get surprised at times.

α_2-Adrenergic agonists can be administered IV, intramuscularly (IM), or subcutaneously (SQ) and produce a dose-dependent degree of sedation, muscle relaxation, and analgesia. Intravenous administration of α_2-adrenergic agonists provides a faster onset and more intense level of chemical restraint and analgesia. The fairly rapid onset time can be used to advantage, allowing multiple smaller IV doses of an α_2-adrenergic agonist to be administered in an attempt to titrate the effect to the desired level. Intramuscular administration results in a more gradual onset and provides a longer duration of less intense chemical restraint and analgesia. Intramuscular administration is often used when patient cooperation does not allow IV administration or when extended duration is desired. The intramuscular dose is traditionally twice the IV dose one would select for the patient based on the desired level of effect and the patient's initial demeanor. SQ administration results in the most gradual onset, longest duration, and mildest peak effect. Administering the IV dose IM or SQ is a method used to produce a degree of sedation with limited the risk for recumbency.

α_2-Adrenergic agonists produce dose-dependent side effects, including decreases in gastrointestinal motility and cardiorespiratory function.[2] α_2-Adrenergic agonists should be avoided or used cautiously in compromised patients and should be reversed on completion of the procedure. Even in normal healthy patients, when large doses of α_2-adrenergic agonists are administered (especially doses used to produce recumbency), reversal is advisable to minimize the risk for gastrointestinal complications. Xylazine has been reported to increase uterine tone in late gestation.[3]

In tractable ruminants the response to xylazine is fairly predictable. Titrated administration (eg, initial conservative dose that is supplemented if necessary) minimizes the incidence of unintended recumbency. Extremely anxious or unruly patients require larger doses of xylazine to achieve adequate control. In these patients the administration process often triggers even greater behavior problems so they should be dosed fairly aggressively at the outset. Intramuscular administration is frequently the only option available in extremely anxious or unruly patients. A calm environment can also help to reduce the dose of xylazine required to calm the patient. Restraint or interaction should be minimized whenever possible until xylazine has produced a reasonable degree of patient control.

Unless contraindicated, anxious or unruly patients should be sedated with xylazine 5 to 10 minutes before the anesthetic induction sequence. The dose of xylazine depends on the demeanor of the patient. It could easily be argued that all healthy ruminant patients might benefit from a small dose of xylazine (0.0075–0.01 mg/kg IV or 0.015–0.02 mg/kg IM) 5 to 10 minutes before anesthetic induction, because even the calmest of patients experience some anxiety from the events surrounding anesthetic induction.

Additional information on the use of sedatives in ruminants can be found in Refs. [1,4].

α_2-Adrenergic Agonist Reversal

Yohimbine or tolazoline may be used to reverse the effects of α_2-adrenergic agonists at the end of a procedure to facilitate a quicker recovery and minimize the risk for gastrointestinal complications. Intramuscular administration of the reversal agent is preferred in all but emergency situations because it decreases the risk for CNS excitement or cardiovascular complications. The shorter duration of action of the reversal agents when given IV can result in resedation in patients when the α_2-adrenergic agonist was administered IM, especially when larger doses were used. Reversal of α_2-adrenergic agonists should not be attempted until sufficient time has elapsed to allow any ketamine or Telazol used to resolve (15–30 minutes post-IV and 30–45 minutes post-IM, respectively) to reduce the chances of a rough recovery. The amount of reversal agent used depends on the dose of the α_2-adrenergic agonist and time since administration. The recommended emergency doses for yohimbine (0.125 mg/kg IV) and tolazoline (2 mg/kg IV) are typically used as the maximum IM dose and reduced to fit the circumstances. When dosed properly the effects of reversal should start to become evident about 10 minutes following IM administration. Splitting the reversal dose (using both IV and IM routes) can produce a quicker recovery while minimizing the risk for resedation. Response to the small IV component is fairly quick, so the primary IM component should be administered first.

Guaifenesin

Guaifenesin is a centrally acting muscle relaxant with mild to moderate sedative activity. At clinically used doses it produces minimal cardiorespiratory effects. Guaifenesin is used in combination with ketamine and in some cases xylazine to produce anesthetic induction in food animal patients. Guaifenesin–ketamine and guaifenesin–ketamine–xylazine combinations are also used in the intravenous maintenance of anesthesia in food animal patients.

Guaifenesin concentrations of 10% have been shown to cause hemolysis in ruminant patients. Practices mixing guaifenesin from powder stock should prepare solutions of 5%. Pre-mixed guaifenesin solution (5%) is now commercially available in 1-L bottles.

Muscle relaxation and ataxia limit the amount of guaifenesin that can be administered before the induction bolus in large patients. In horses guaifenesin is typically preceded by xylazine, which also produces muscle relaxation and ataxia. The typical equine induction sequence delivers 40 to 50 mg/kg of guaifenesin. Anesthetic induction of small ruminants with Double Drip typically delivers 100 mg/kg. In larger cattle administration of Double Drip immediately preceding the induction bolus typically delivers 30 mg/kg.

Anesthetic Agents

Ketamine, tiletamine, and the ultra-short barbiturate thiopental are the injectable anesthetic agents used in large animal practice. Ketamine is by far the most common injectable anesthetic agent used in large animal practice. Thiopental is no longer generally used in large animal practice for induction or maintenance of anesthesia, but remains the fastest option for restoring an anesthetized state when larger ruminant patients get too light during inhalation of maintenance anesthesia. Thiopental (1.1 mg/kg IV) is also useful in dulling the protective swallowing reflex present during ketamine-based injectable anesthesia. Tiletamine, a more potent and longer-lasting relative of ketamine, is available only in combination with the benzodiazepine zolazepam as Telazol. Because of the high cost of Telazol, it is primarily used in large animal practice for capturing "wild" patients.[4]

Ketamine and tiletamine draw on sympathetic nervous system reserve to augment cardiac output and blood pressure. This effect helps counter their direct negative inotropic and vasodilatory effects and the negative cardiovascular effects produced by xylazine. Cardiovascular function in normal healthy patients anesthetized with ketamine-based protocols is good to excellent. I cannot emphasize enough the need for caution in dosing these seemingly safe drugs in compromised patients in which sympathetic reserve may be severely limited.

ANESTHETIC TECHNIQUES

Ketamine Stun

Ketamine is a dissociative anesthetic commonly used in veterinary medicine. Ketamine possesses potent analgesic effects when administered at subanesthetic doses. Adding a small dose of ketamine to more traditional chemical restraint combinations greatly enhances the level of patient cooperation. This technique is called the "ketamine stun" (or "stun") because of the stunned effect it produces in patients when administered IV at doses that produce recumbency. These patients appear to be awake, but seem oblivious to surroundings and procedures being performed. The IV effect is brief (approximately 15 minutes) and patients typically stand and appear fairly normal at that time. I initially referred to this state as semianesthetized, but perhaps chemical hypnosis is more appropriate. The ketamine stun technique makes treating camelid patients, which are frequently uncooperative, much more pleasant.[5] Because of the success in camelid patients the stun technique was adjusted for use in small ruminants (less xylazine) and proved to be just as useful. Dosing must be more conservative when using the ketamine stun technique in standing patients. This practice limits the degree of systemic analgesia relative to what we can achieve in recumbent patients, but still provides improved patient cooperation when compared with more traditional methods of standing chemical restraint in ruminants and horses.

The stun is basically the addition of a small dose of ketamine to any chemical restraint technique. In ruminants and camelid patients a combination of xylazine, butorphanol, and ketamine is typically used. In equine patients I generally use detomidine, morphine, and ketamine. Morphine (0.05–0.06 mg/kg) has been substituted in some ruminant stuns. Morphine is much cheaper than butorphanol. In standing adult cattle stuns a similar level of cooperation is achieved with either opioid, but patients seem less obtunded when morphine is used. Some practitioners may find the obtunded appearance useful because it allows them to follow the decay over time in the level of chemical restraint. Morphine is used to provide analgesic relief in food animal patients. More information of the use of morphine in ruminants can be found in Ref. [6].

α_2-Adrenergic agonists possess potent sedative and analgesic effects. Opioids are typically thought of as analgesic drugs, but they possess CNS effects that when combined with tranquilizers or sedatives produce a greater level of mental depression. Ketamine is an N-methyl-D-aspartate receptor antagonist that possesses potent analgesic effects at subanesthetic doses. Ketamine was initially included in the stun technique for its analgesic properties, but it likely contributes to the mental aspects of the enhanced cooperation exhibited by patients under the influence of the ketamine stun technique. By combining drugs clinicians are able to use smaller oses of the individual components while still achieving the desired level of effect.

Ketamine stun techniques can be divided into two broad categories, standing and recumbent. The standing ketamine stun is used primarily in large ruminants and horses. The recumbent ketamine stun is used primarily in small ruminants, camelids, and foals. The level of effect achieved is determined by three variables (dose, route of administration, initial demeanor of the patient). The stun cocktail can be administered IV, IM, or SQ, depending on the systemic analgesia, patient cooperation, and duration desired (**Table 1**).

Aggressive dosing increases the level of systemic analgesia and patient cooperation, but also increases duration of recumbency or the risk for unintended recumbency. Xylazine is the most variable component of the stun combination. Initial patient demeanor plays a large role in the effect obtained from xylazine administration. Response to xylazine in tractable ruminants is fairly predictable. To minimize the incidence of unintended recumbency a titrated approach (eg, initial conservative dose that is supplemented if necessary) should be used. Extremely anxious or unruly patients require larger doses of xylazine to achieve adequate control. In these patients the administration process often triggers even greater behavior problems so they should be dosed fairly aggressively at the outset.

Many permutations are possible when using the ketamine stun. Several years of experimentation in many different species has provided me with a great deal of insight into the potential of this technique, but has not produced a definitive combination for all situations in each species. The following examples are provided as a guide and practitioners are encouraged to experiment with adjustments in doses. I would like to thank Dr. David Anderson, who has used the ketamine stun technique extensively in food animal patients at Kansas State University, for his support during the development of the technique and his contributions to this section.

Clinical application of the ketamine stun in food animal patients can be divided into four basic categories.

Table 1
Route of administration determines the relative impact of the ketamine stun technique

Parameter	Relative Ranking
Intensity (analgesia/cooperation)	IV >> IM > SQ
Onset	IV >> IM > SQ
Duration of effect	SQ > IM >> IV

Intravenous recumbent stun

The IV recumbent stun is used for short procedures or procedures requiring a high level of systemic analgesia and patient cooperation.

A combination of xylazine (0.025–0.05 mg/kg), butorphanol (0.05–0.1 mg/kg), and ketamine (0.3–0.5 mg/kg) is administered IV. Onset is approximately 1 minute. Patients gracefully become recumbent. Patients appear to be awake, but seem oblivious to surroundings and procedures being performed. Mild random head or limb motion is not unusual, but purposeful movement or vocalization are signs of an inadequate stun level and additional drug should be administered. Half of the initial ketamine dose should be administered IV and is often effective. If, after allowing 60 to 90 seconds for onset, this additional half dose of ketamine fails to produce the desired level of analgesia a second half dose of ketamine along with half of the initial dose of xylazine should be administered IV. The level of systemic analgesia produced varies depending on the doses administered, but tends to be fairly intense. Surgical levels of analgesia have been achieved with this technique, but local anesthetic blockade should be used whenever feasible to reduce the risk for patient awareness and stress. Duration of the stun effect is approximately 15 minutes and patients typically are able to stand and walk immediately or shortly after this point. The IV recumbent stun is designed for short procedures. The clinician should plan ahead and work quickly. Supplemental doses of ketamine or xylazine can be administered to extend duration, but this technique is not intended for procedures that are expected to last significantly beyond the 15- to 25-minute range. The degree of extension is relative to the amount of supplemental drug administered.

The recumbent IV stun has proved useful for facilitating short procedures in camelids and small ruminants.

Intramuscular or subcutaneous recumbent stun

The IM or SQ recumbent stun is used for procedures requiring a longer duration of chemical restraint. The level of systemic analgesia is not as intense and local anesthetic blockade should be used to reduce the risk for patient awareness and stress. Umbilical hernia repair is an example of the procedures performed using this technique. This approach is also useful for improving cooperation in patients that have gone down before or during a surgical procedure.

A combination of butorphanol (0.025 mg/kg), xylazine (0.05 mg/kg), and ketamine (0.1 mg/kg) is administered IM or SQ. SQ administration is preferred because it provides a slightly longer duration of effect. Onset time is approximately 3 to 10 minutes. Patients are obtunded enough to require (and tolerate) intubation when placed in dorsal recumbency. Information on intubating and positioning patients to promote saliva egress can be found in Ref. [1]. Duration of effect with SQ administration is approximately 45 minutes. Patients should be ambulatory within 30 minutes following this point.

The level of systemic analgesia produced by the IM or SQ recumbent stun is not as intense, but this approach provides an enhanced level of patient cooperation that can make procedures much more pleasant for patient and clinician.

Intravenous standing stun

The IV standing stun is typically used to provide a transient improvement in patient cooperation. Small IV boluses of ketamine have also been used to provide short periods of enhanced analgesia in equine colic patients.[7] Xylazine (0.02–0.0275 mg/kg), butorphanol (0.02–0.1 mg/kg, see later discussion), and ketamine (0.05–0.1 mg/kg) can be administered individually or as a combination.

An example of the effectiveness of the IV standing stun technique is a 725 to 775 kg Charolais bull that was run into the chute for examination of a possible penile injury. He was extremely agitated and kept banging around inside the chute despite being left alone. Examination was impossible and patient injury was a valid concern. To calm him down, I administered 20 mg of IV xylazine (0.0275 mg/kg). This dose made him stand still when left alone, but he would not tolerate attempts to examine him. I then administered 40 mg of IV ketamine (0.055 mg/kg). The ketamine made him extremely cooperative, but the chute hampered full examination. A decision to place him on the tilt table was made. He was compliant during the tabling process and subsequent examination. Intravenous ketamine boluses typically last approximately 15 minutes, although patients may remain more cooperative beyond this point when using the IV stun technique.

Small doses of IV ketamine can markedly improve the degree of patient cooperation in standing chemical restraint. Butorphanol (0.05–0.1 mg/kg IV or IM in smaller ruminants, 0.02–0.05 mg/kg IV or IM in larger ruminants) or morphine (0.05–0.1 mg/kg IV or IM) can be added to augment the level of analgesia and patient control.

Intramuscular or subcutaneous standing stun

5–10–20 technique The IM or SQ standing stun is used for most standing procedures in ruminant patients. The level of systemic analgesia is limited and local anesthetic blockade should be used to reduce the risk for patient awareness and stress. Standing flank laparotomy is an example of the procedures performed using this technique.

In beef cattle a combination of butorphanol (0.01 mg/kg), xylazine (0.02 mg/kg), and ketamine (0.04 mg/kg) is administered IM or SQ. In a 500-kg cow this equates to butorphanol (5 mg), xylazine (10 mg), and ketamine (20 mg). For a 680-kg patient the doses are 7 mg butorphanol, 15 mg xylazine, and 25 mg ketamine. Dosages may need to be adjusted when using the IM/SQ stun technique in milder mannered cattle.

The 5 mg–10 mg–20 mg combination has been used in student junior surgery laboratories at Kansas State to provide chemical restraint for standing cesarean sections in beef cattle. Patient weights varied from 340 to 660 kg, but no adjustments were made in the combination administered. SQ administration is preferred to minimize the risk for recumbency. In unruly cows IM administration provides better patient control. Onset is 5 to 10 minutes with SQ administration. The initial dose of 5–10–20 did not result in recumbency. Cows stood quietly during the cesarean sections (many were ill mannered before the ketamine stun). Duration of effect is approximately 60 to 90 minutes. Additional xylazine and ketamine can be administered SQ to extend the duration of chemical restraint. Recumbency has occasionally occurred with re-administration of 50% of all three components. Current recommendation for supplemental drug administration is 25% to 50% of the initial Xylazine and ketamine doses (0–2.5–5) and (0–5–10), respectively, depending on the degree of cooperation and time required to complete the procedure.

A similar approach (10–20–40 technique) has been used successfully in adult bulls. Preputial surgery (with a local anesthetic block) is an example of the procedures performed using this technique.

The IM/SQ standing stun is a simple method for improving the quality of standing procedures for patient and clinician.

Intravenous Xylazine–Ketamine

Intravenous xylazine and ketamine can be used to produce a short duration of injectable anesthesia in normal healthy ruminants. Because of the large dose of xylazine this technique should not be used in compromised patients.

Xylazine (0.05 mg/kg IV) is administered first. When marked sedation is evident or the patient becomes recumbent, ketamine (2 mg/kg IV) is administered. This combination provides approximately 15 minutes of anesthesia. Administration of one third to one half of the original dose of each drug can be used to extend anesthesia, but recovery duration increases with the number of supplemental doses administered because of the slower clearance of xylazine. Gradually reducing the xylazine component in the supplemental doses reduces its adverse impact on cardiorespiratory function and recovery time. Extending anesthesia with boluses of IV xylazine–ketamine should be limited to cases that require only a few supplemental doses or in emergency situations in which other options are not available. Double Drip or Ruminant Triple Drip are the preferred methods for extending the duration of injectable anesthesia in ruminant patients. Cardiorespiratory function is good to excellent with this combination in normal, healthy ruminant patients. Recovery quality is good.

Intramuscular Xylazine–Ketamine

Intramuscular administration of xylazine and ketamine can be used to produce an intermediate length of injectable anesthesia in normal healthy ruminants. Because of the large dose of xylazine this technique should not be used in compromised patients.

A combination of xylazine (0.05–0.1 mg/kg IM) and ketamine (4 mg/kg IM) is administered. This combination generally produces 30 to 40 minutes of recumbency. As with any bolus administration technique analgesia is highest at the outset and gradually diminishes over time. A half dose of each drug can be administered IM to extend duration 15 to 20 minutes. A quarter dose of each drug can be administered IV to extend duration of anesthesia approximately 10 to 15 minutes. Cardiorespiratory function is good to excellent with this combination in normal, healthy ruminant patients. Recovery quality is good.

Butorphanol–Ketamine–Xylazine

The butorphanol–ketamine–xylazine technique was developed by Dr. LaRue Johnson at Colorado State University. He prefers to call it XKB, but everyone else refers to it as BKX. A combination of xylazine, ketamine, and butorphanol is administered IM to produce an intermediate duration of injectable anesthesia in normal healthy ruminants. Because of the large dose of xylazine this technique should not be used in compromised patients.

A stock solution can be created to provide numerous doses by adding 100 mg of large animal xylazine (1 mL) and 10 mg of butorphanol (1 mL) to a bottle of ketamine (1000 mg). Administer the mixture IM at a dose rate of 1 mL/20 kg. An alternative method is to draw up the individual components in a syringe as follows:

Butorphanol (0.0375 mg/kg);
Xylazine (0.375 mg/kg);
Ketamine (3.75 mg/kg).

The patient should become recumbent within 3 to 5 minutes with a surgical plane of anesthesia lasting up to another 20 to 30 minutes. As with any bolus administration technique analgesia is highest at the outset and gradually diminishes over time. For procedures requiring considerable surgical preparation the effective period of analgesia can be extended by administering half of the initial BKX dose IV before the start of surgery. Expect approximately 25 to 35 minutes of working time when the additional dose is used. Patients tend to remain laterally recumbent much longer following completion of the procedure when compared with the recumbent ketamine stun techniques. Cardiorespiratory function is good to excellent with this combination in normal, healthy ruminant patients. Recovery quality is good.

Ruminant Triple Drip

Ruminant Triple Drip is created by adding ketamine (1 mg/mL) and xylazine (0.1 mg/mL) to 5% guaifenesin.[8,9] Equine Triple Drip has a much higher concentration of xylazine (0.5 mg/mL). A constant-rate infusion of Ruminant Triple Drip can be used to provide a stable plane of injectable anesthesia in normal healthy ruminants. Compromised ruminant patients should be maintained with Double Drip to eliminate the cardiovascular depressant effects of xylazine.

In small ruminants anesthetic induction is achieved by slowly infusing Ruminant Triple Drip to effect. A syringe should be used to administer Ruminant Triple Drip in small patients to reduce the risk for overdosing because this combination has a somewhat slow onset. Muscle relaxation and sedation typically produce recumbency well before the patient is anesthetized. Anesthetic induction generally requires administration of 1.0 to 1.5 mL/kg. Anesthesia can be maintained in normal healthy ruminants by continued infusion of Ruminant Triple Drip at a rate of 2.5 mL/kg/h without significant cardiorespiratory depression. Xylazine is cleared more slowly than ketamine. Because of this difference postprocedure recumbency lengthens as the duration of Ruminant Triple Drip administration increases. Xylazine sedation can be reversed to speed the recovery process once the patient is awake. Recovery quality is good.

In large ruminants Double Drip is generally used to soften up the patient, but Triple Drip could also be used for this purpose. When early signs of sedation and muscle relaxation become evident, a combination of ketamine (1.5–2 mg/kg IV) and diazepam (0.06–0.1 mg/kg IV) is administered. This approach provides a more predictable and rapid drop, improving patient control and safety of personnel involved in the induction process. Anesthesia can be maintained with continued infusion of either Double Drip or Ruminant Triple Drip. Cardiorespiratory function is good to excellent with this approach in normal, healthy large ruminant patients. Recovery quality is good.

Double Drip

Double Drip is created by adding ketamine (1 mg/mL) to 5% guaifenesin. Double Drip is the most commonly used method for inducing anesthesia to be maintained with inhalants in small ruminants. A constant-rate infusion of Double Drip can be used to provide a stable plane of injectable anesthesia in ruminants. Because Double Drip does not contain xylazine the level of analgesia provided is somewhat lower when compared with Ruminant Triple Drip. The absence of xylazine's cardiovascular depressant effects makes Double Drip a better choice for injectable maintenance in compromised ruminant patients. Butorphanol (0.05–0.1 mg/kg IV or IM in smaller ruminants, 0.02–0.05 mg/kg IV or IM in larger ruminants) or morphine (0.05–0.1 mg/kg IV or IM) can be administered to augment the level of analgesia when Double Drip is used to maintain anesthesia.

Anesthetic induction is achieved by slowly administering Double Drip to effect. A syringe should be used to administer Double Drip in small patients to reduce the risk for overdosing because this combination has a somewhat slow onset. Muscle relaxation and sedation typically produce recumbency well before the patient is anesthetized. Anesthetic induction generally requires administration of 1.5 to 2.0 mL/kg. Anesthesia can be maintained by continued infusion of Double Drip at a rate of approximately 2.5 mL/kg/h without significant cardiorespiratory depression in normal healthy patients. In compromised patients sympathetic nervous system reserve may be limited. Although Double Drip is the most benign method of injectable anesthesia, care must be taken to minimize anesthetic depth in severely compromised patients. Cardiorespiratory function should be monitored and supportive measures (IV fluids, dobutamine, oxygen, and so forth) implemented as required. Recovery quality is good.

For large ruminants refer to Ruminant Triple Drip section.

Ketamine–Diazepam

Intravenous diazepam and ketamine (Ket–Val) can be used to produce a short duration of injectable anesthesia in normal healthy ruminants. Cardiovascular function is good to excellent following induction with this combination in normal healthy patients and the absence of xylazine's cardiovascular depressant effects makes Ket–Val a viable choice for injectable anesthesia of compromised patients. The same admonitions provided for Double Drip should be applied when using Ket–Val to anesthetize severely compromised patients. Titrated administration can be used to minimize the level of effect produced when administering boluses of Ket–Val. Butorphanol (0.05–0.1 mg/kg IV or IM in smaller ruminants, 0.02–0.05 mg/kg IV or IM in larger ruminants), or morphine (0.05–0.1 mg/kg IV or IM) can be administered to augment the level of analgesia when using Ket–Val to anesthetize ruminant patients.

In small ruminants a mixture of equal volumes of ketamine (100 mg/mL) and diazepam (5 mg/mL) is administered intravenously at 1 mL/18–22 kg (which sounded better when it was 1 mL/40–50 lb). A single bolus of Ket–Val provides up to 15 to 20 minutes of surgical analgesia with patients remaining recumbent somewhat longer. As with any bolus administration technique analgesia is highest at the outset and gradually diminishes over time. Administering smaller boluses (one third to one half of the original volume) can be used to extend anesthetic duration. Anesthesia can also be maintained with IV infusion of either Double Drip or Ruminant Triple Drip, which provides a more stable plane of anesthesia than intermittent boluses of Ket–Val. Recovery quality is good.

For large ruminants refer to Ruminant Triple Drip section.

REFERENCES

1. Abrahamsen EJ. Inhalation anesthesia in ruminants. In: Anderson DE, Rings M, editors. Current Veterinary Therapy Food Animal Practice. 5th edition. Saunders/Elsevier; 2009. p. 559–69.
2. Campbell KB, Klavano PA, Richardson P, et al. Hemodynamic effects of xylazine in the calf. Am J Vet Res 1979;40:1777–80.
3. LeBlanc MM, Hubbell JAE, Smith HC. The effects of xylazine hydrochloride on intrauterine pressure in the cow and the mare. Theriogenology 1984;21(5):681–90.
4. Abrahamsen EJ. Chemical restraint in ruminants. Vet Clin North Am Food Anim Pract 2008;24(2):227–43.
5. Abrahamsen EJ. Sedation/chemical restraint/anesthesia. Presented at the Proceedings of the 2004, 2006, 2008 International Camelid Health Conference for veterinarians. Columbus (OH), March 2004, 2006, 2008.

6. Abrahamsen EJ. Managing severe pain in ruminants. In: Anderson DE, Rings M, editors. Current Veterinary Therapy Food Animal Practice. 5th edition. Saunders/Elsevier; 2009. p. 570–4.
7. Abrahamsen EJ. How to medicate a horse with colic before referral. In: Proceedings of the 2005 British Equine Veterinary Association (BEVA) Congress. Harrogate (England), September 2005. p. 45–6.
8. Lin HC, Tyler JW, Welles EG, et al. Effects of anesthesia induced and maintained by continuous intravenous administration of guaifenesin, ketamine, and xylazine in spontaneously breathing sheep. Am J Vet Res 1993;54(11):1913–6.
9. Thurmon JC, Benson GJ, Tranquilli WJ, et al. Cardiovascular effects of intravenous infusion of guaifenesin, ketamine, and xylazine in Holstein calves. Vet Surg 1986; 15:463.

Development of Teaser Bulls Under Field Conditions

Gregor L. Morgan, BVSc, MS, PhD[a,*], Lionel J. Dawson, BVSc, MS[a,b]

KEYWORDS

• Sterilization • Surgery • Bulls • Teaser • Field conditions

A major contributing factor to the successful outcome of an artificial insemination program in cattle is accurate identification of "in estrus" female animals, which, in turn, facilitates accurate timing of insemination. In addition to visual observation, numerous aids are available to assist in heat detection. These include tail head paints or crayons, glue-on dye patches (KAMAR heat mount detectors), self-adhesive patches (Estrotect-Estrus Alert), and electronic pressure-sensitive mount detectors (Heat-Watch). Each of these aids has its advantages and disadvantages but all rely on the "in estrus" female animal to stand and be ridden by others in the herd.[1–3] A more natural situation is to use an intact but sterilized bull, often referred to as a teaser bull, to aid in heat detection. These animals are more likely to identify truly "in estrus" female animals and those with short and or weak estrus expression. If turned out before the breeding season, they may also be used to hasten the onset of cycling in peripubertal heifers and shorten the postcalving anestrus period in lactating beef cows.[3]

The three objectives in the surgical preparation of a teaser bull are first, to render him sterile, second, to prevent venereal disease transmission, and third, to avoid diminished libido so the bull will remain active for a long period of time.[4]

Two surgical procedures that will not prevent intromission, but will sterilize the bull are vasectomy and caudal epididymectomy. In some "closed herds," either of these procedures is done to create a teaser bull but they provide no protection against venereal disease transmission. Creating teaser bulls from within the home herd does not protect against a neighborhood bull infected with a venereal disease breaking through boundary fences and infecting a naive herd. Therefore, it is strongly recommended that one of several surgical procedures be done which prevents intromission. Indeed, at this time, this recommendation is appropriate, given the increasing number of beef herds found to be infected with *Tritrichomonas fetus* in the United States.

[a] Center for Veterinary Health Sciences, Oklahoma State University, 1-BVMTH, Room 002, Stillwater, OK 74078, USA
[b] American Institute for Goat Research, Langston University, Langston, OK 73050, USA
* Corresponding author.
E-mail address: gregor.morgan@okstate.edu (G.L. Morgan).

Vet Clin Food Anim 24 (2008) 443–453
doi:10.1016/j.cvfa.2008.06.004
vetfood.theclinics.com
0749-0720/08/$ – see front matter © 2008 Elsevier Inc. All rights reserved.

Surgical procedures that prevent intromission fall into one of two categories:

1. Those that allow protrusion but not intromission (penile-prepuce translocation [PPT])
2. Those that prevent penile protrusion, thereby preventing intromission (penopexy)

GUIDELINES FOR SELECTING AN APPROPRIATE BULL

Only intact bulls can be surgically modified to make a teaser animal, which stems from a past practice of using several growth implants in the ear or injections of long-acting testosterone products to steers, nonreplacement heifers, freemartins, or cull cows. This practice today is clearly a violation of the Animal Medicinal Drug Use Clarification Act (AMDUCA) and therefore is illegal. For the most part, these practices resulted in effective teaser animals and if female animals were used, surgical procedures to prevent intromission were not needed. However, because the practice is illegal, it will not be discussed further.

Bulls to be prepared as teasers should be selected well before the breeding season to allow time for healing and continued growth. They should be of mild temperament to facilitate handling, be of moderate adult size, and have strong libido. The last is difficult to predict in young bulls. Regardless of the surgical procedure chosen, all are more easily performed on bulls weighing less than 600 pounds. Large bulls are more difficult to manage physically, tend to hemorrhage more, take longer to complete the surgical procedure, and tend to have more postsurgical complications.

FIELD RESTRAINT FOR SURGERY

The required restraint depends on facilities available, size and demeanor of the bull, procedure to be performed, and available help. Numerous drug protocols can be used for sedation or general anesthesia (GA). For sterilization purposes, vasectomy and caudal epididymectomy may be performed with standing sedation and local lidocaine line block over the surgery site. A tail jack may be a useful additional restraint. Practitioners have their own preferences with respect to sedation or GA under field conditions. Nevertheless, **Table 1** presents several drug protocols for sedation or GA that have been used by the authors.

For sedation purposes, xylazine is commonly used at a dose range of 0.05 to 0.1 mg/kg intramuscularly or intravenously However, under most circumstances, a more invasive surgery is performed in addition to sterilization to prevent intromission, and the preferred procedures may require GA. Under field conditions, GA can be difficult and is not without risk to surgeon and patient. However, proper preparation will minimize complications. Bulls in the 600 lb or less range are preferred. Feed should be withheld from the bull 48 hours and water 12 hours before surgery.

PREFERRED SURGICAL PROCEDURES USED TO CREATE TEASER BULLS

Several techniques are described in the literature for preparing a teaser bull. This article discusses those more preferred by the authors and that may be done in a field situation.

Vasectomy

This procedure may be done standing in a chute with mild sedation and local anesthesia over the surgical site, or the animal may be restrained in right lateral or dorsal recumbency using heavy sedation and ropes. With the bull standing, the approach from

Table 1
Anesthetic protocols used successfully in bulls under field conditions

Drug	Dosage	Route	Duration
Standing sedation with mild analgesia			
Xylazine	0.05–0.10 mg/kg	IV or IM Lower dose IV	15–30 min
Xylazine	0.02–0.03 mg/kg With lidocaine	Caudal epidural	15–30 min
Mild sedation with good analgesia			
Ketamine	Butorphanol, 0.025 mg/kg; xylazine, 0.050 mg/kg; ketamine, 0.100 mg/kg	IV	<30 min
—	Double the dose	IM	<30 min
Recumbent sedation with analgesia			
Xylazine–ketamine	Xylazine, 0.05 mg/kg; wait 5 min; ketamine, 2–4mg/kg	IV IV	30–45 min
—	Xylazine, 0.10 mg/kg; wait 10–15 min; ketamine 2–4 mg/kg	IM IV or IM	30–45 min
Xylazine–telazol	Xylazine, 0.05–0.10 mg/kg; Telazol, 4–5 mg/kg	IM IM	60–75 min
Triple drip 1-L bottle of guaifenesin + 1000 mg ketamine + 100 mg xylazine	Induction: 0.5–1.0 mL/kg; maintenance: 2 mL/kg	IV IV	75–90 min

Tolazoline, an alpha2-adrenergic receptor antagonist, may be used to reverse the effects of xylazine, 2mg/kg, IV or IM.
Abbreviations: IM, intramuscular; IV, intravenous.

the anterior aspect of the scrotal neck can be difficult because of limited access and therefore, the posterior approach is recommended for vasectomy. In either position, the neck of the scrotum is clipped and prepped for aseptic surgery. Local anesthetic is injected along two proposed incision lines over each spermatic cord or along a single incision approach over the median raphe of the scrotum beginning 6 to 8 cm above each testicle.[5,6]

A 3-cm incision is made through the skin and tunica dartos to expose the spermatic cord within the tunica vaginalis (**Fig. 1**). The ductus deferens (DD) is readily identified by palpating a firm cord-like structure approximately 2 to 3 mm in diameter in the spermatic cord. The cord is carefully dissected free of surrounding tissue and a curved hemostat is placed under the cord to elevate it through the skin incision (**Fig. 2**). A 2- to 3-cm incision is made through the tunica vaginalis in an area not covered by the cremaster muscle to expose the contents and identify the vas deferens. Great care must be taken with this incision to avoid cutting the pampiniform plexus or other structures within the cord. Once the DD is identified, two ligatures are placed around it approximately 3 to 5 cm apart using #0 absorbable suture. The DD between the ligatures is removed and the skin closed with a nonabsorbable suture (**Fig. 3**).[5,6] The

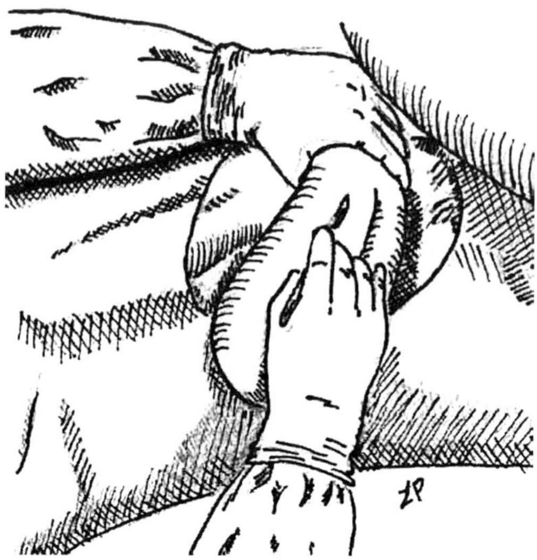

Fig. 1. A 3-cm skin incision made in the scrotal neck and continued deeper through the tunica dartos exposing the spermatic cord.

excised DD is taken and the contents squeezed onto a slide and observed under a microscope for spermatozoa. Postsurgical antibiotics may be given to guard against infection at the surgical site and the bull may take up to 30 days to clear all sperm from the system so he should not be used until this time guideline has been met.

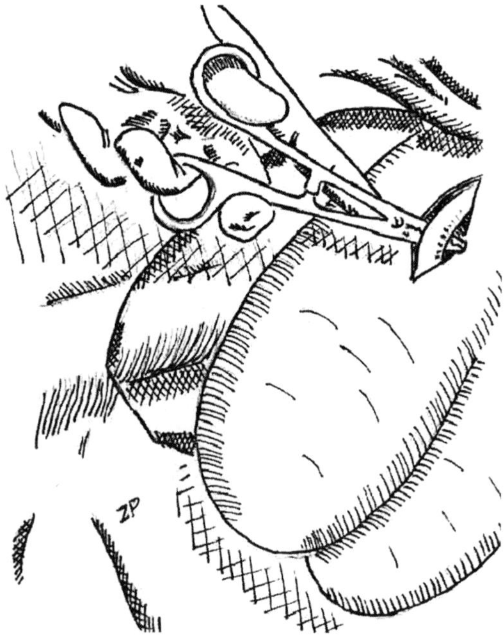

Fig. 2. Spermatic cord freed from the surrounding tissue, elevated with hemostats and carefully opened.

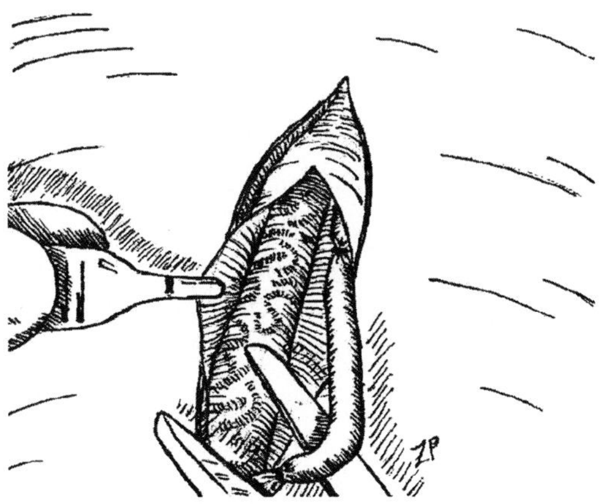

Fig. 3. The DD is isolated and two ligatures, 2 to 3 cm apart, and the segment, are removed.

Caudal Epididymectomy

This procedure is preferred over a vasectomy because it is simpler and can be performed with the patient lightly sedated in a standing position. The area of the scrotum over the tail of the epididymis is clipped, surgically prepped, and infiltrated with a local anesthetic. The surgeon then grasps the neck of the scrotum over one testicle, forcing it ventrally. A 2- to 3-cm skin incision is made directly over the tail of the epididymis, parallel to the raphe (**Fig. 4**).The incision is continued through the common vaginal tunic until the tail of the epididymis "pops out." With careful dissection, the tail of the epididymis is freed from the testicle and an Allis tissue forceps is used to grasp and exteriorize the tail of the epididymis fully. The DD and the body of the epididymis are identified and each is clamped by a hemostat. A nonabsorbable suture is placed proximal to each clamp and the tail of the epididymis is removed (**Fig. 5**). This procedure is repeated on the other testicle. The common vaginal tunic is closed with an absorbable simple interrupted suture pattern, whereas the skin on the scrotum may be left open (**Fig. 6**).[4–14] A postsurgical antibiotic is not necessary if the animal is put in

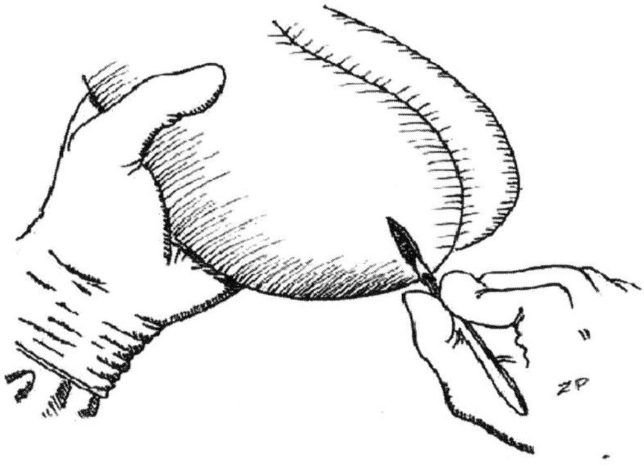

Fig. 4. The testicle is forced to the bottom of the scrotum, the tail of the epididymis is identified, and an incision is made directly over the tail. The incision is continued deeper until the epididymal tail "pops" out.

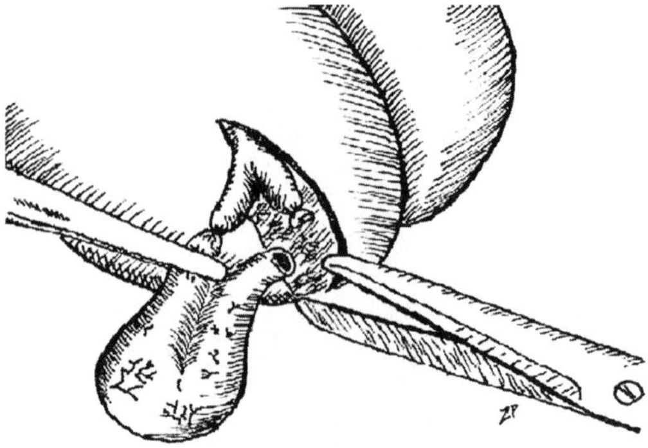

Fig. 5. With careful dissection, the loop formed by the vas deferens and the epididymal tail is identified and ligated on both sides of the loop. The tail is then excised. (*Modified from* Hendrickson DA, editor. Techniques in large animal surgery. 3rd edition. Ames (IA): Blackwell Publishing; 2007. p. 251–6; with permission.)

a clean, dry pen for 5 days after surgery to monitor any abnormal swelling and bleeding.

Penile-Prepuce Translocation

PPT is a surgical procedure that moves the penis and prepuce off the midline to an area in the lower left flank. Protrusion of the penis is not prevented but intromission

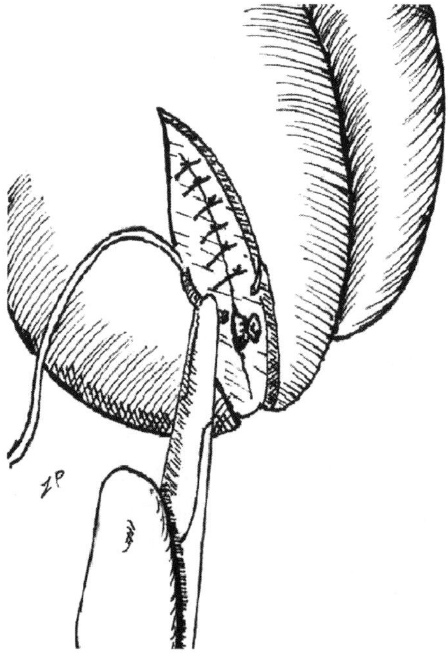

Fig. 6. The common vaginal tunic is closed with absorbable suture material and the skin incision can be left open. (*Modified from* Hendrickson DA, editor. Techniques in large animal surgery. 3rd edition. Ames (IA): Blackwell Publishing; 2007. p. 251–6; with permission.)

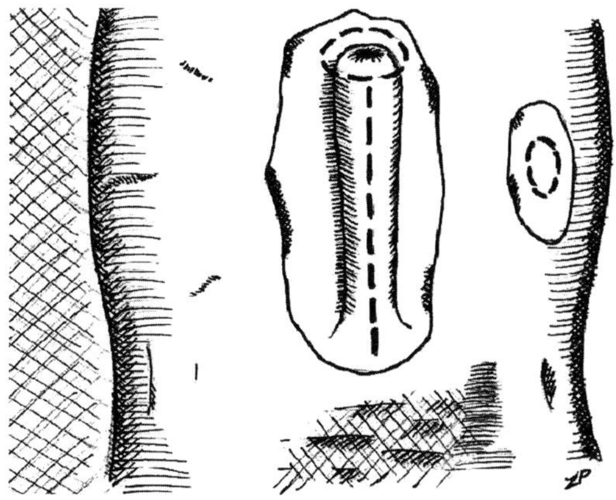

Fig. 7. Outlining of the skin incisions of the penile translocation techniques. (*Modified from* Hendrickson DA, editor. Techniques in large animal surgery. 3rd edition. Ames (IA): Blackwell Publishing; 2007. p. 251–6; with permission.)

is. This procedure is more complicated than other teaser surgeries but, in the authors' opinion, is the preferred technique. These bulls appear to maintain libido and function for a long time, which could be related to the fact that presumably no pain is experienced when they get an erection compared with penile tie-down procedures.

PPT is performed with the patient in dorsal recumbency under GA. The site to which the preputial orifice is to be moved should be marked while the bull is standing normally because it can become distorted when he is in dorsal recumbency and may result in the bull being able to gain intromission. This circular excision of skin should be on the left flank such that the lower edge of the circular excision of skin is 3 cm above the left flank fold.

The surgical area around the preputial orifice to the scrotum and the ventral abdomen on the left are prepared for aseptic surgery.

A single interrupted suture is placed at the dorsal aspect of the preputial orifice to serve as a reference when orienting the orifice into the translocation site. Initially, a circumferential skin incision beginning 4 cm from the preputial orifice is made around the

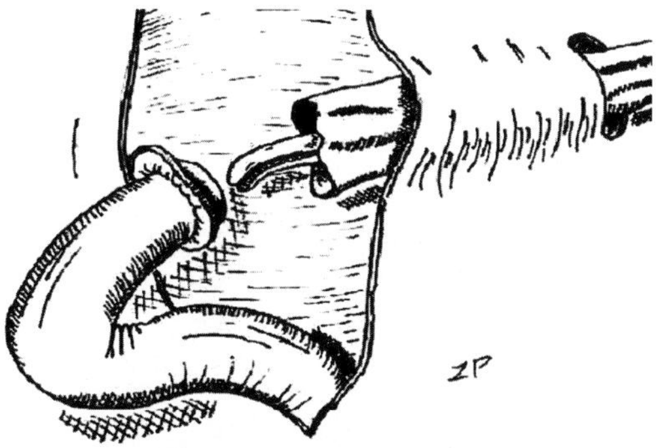

Fig. 8. Subcutaneous tunnel to draw the freed penis-prepuce through to new translocation site. (*Modified from* Hendrickson DA, editor. Techniques in large animal surgery. 3rd edition. Ames (IA): Blackwell Publishing; 2007. p. 251–6; with permission.)

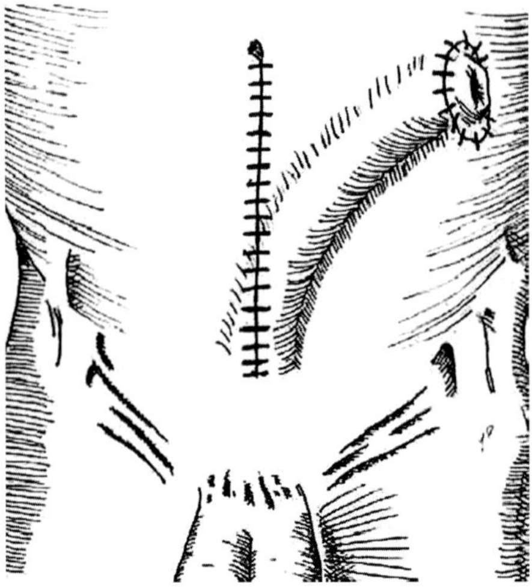

Fig. 9. Translocated penis-prepuce. (*Modified from* Hendrickson DA, editor. Techniques in large animal surgery. 3rd edition. Ames (IA): Blackwell Publishing; 2007. p. 251–6; with permission.)

prepuce and a second midline incision starting cranial to the scrotum is made forward, connecting to the circumferential incision around the preputial opening (**Fig. 7**). The prepuce is carefully dissected free off the abdominal wall, preserving the large blood vessels as much as possible. Significant hemorrhage may occur when dissecting the preputial orifice free from the body wall and must be controlled.

A circular flank incision is made at the previously identified location above the left flank. The diameter of this incision should be similar to the preputial orifice being translocated. After removing the circular piece of skin, a tunnel is made subcutaneously by introducing long sponge forceps or Knowles cervical forceps through the circular flank incision to the caudal end of the midline incision. The tunnel is opened further by opening the forceps sufficiently to redirect the prepuce and penis without any restrictions. A sterile plastic sleeve is placed over the preputial orifice to prevent contamination of the tunnel when the penis and prepuce are pulled through (**Fig. 8**).

Using the previously placed skin suture as a guide, the dorsum of the preputial orifice is aligned with the dorsal aspect of the circular flank incision. The orifice is sutured in two layers. The subcutaneous layer is closed with a simple interrupted pattern using absorbable suture and the skin is closed with a simple interrupted nonabsorbable

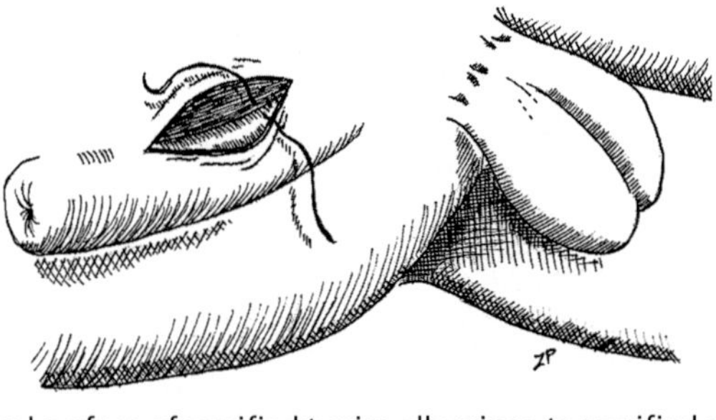

Fig. 10. Suturing dorsal surface of scarified tunica albuginea to scarified surface of linea alba.

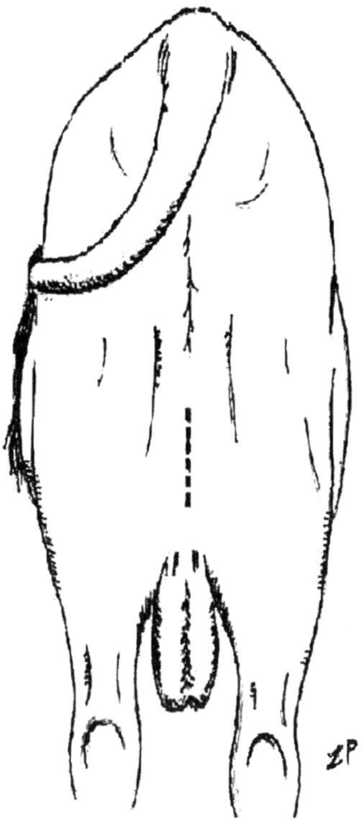

Fig. 11. Incision site for perineal fixation of the penis.

suture (**Fig. 9**). The ventral midline incision is also closed in two layers in a subcutaneous continuous pattern using absorbable suture and incorporating the abdominal fascia to reduce tissue dead space. The skin is closed using nonabsorbable suture in a continuous forward interlocking pattern (see **Fig. 9**). The circular incision at the

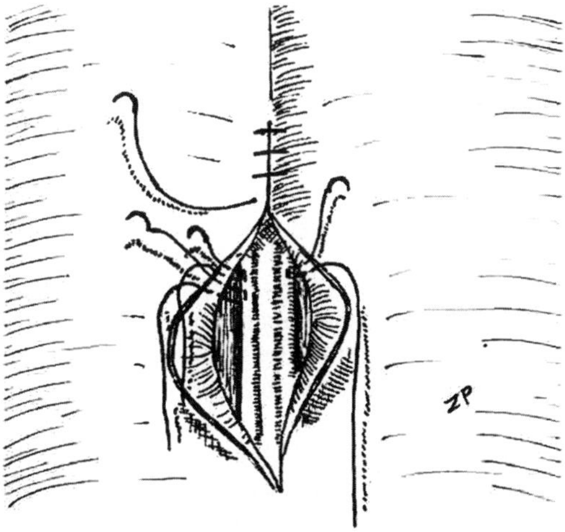

Fig. 12. Preplaced fixation sutures through the tunica albuginea laterally to the subcutaneous fascia.

original preputial opening site is left open for drainage. A bilateral caudal epididymectomy is performed, the bull is administered antibiotics for 5 days, and sutures are removed in 2 weeks. Postoperatively, it is important to make sure the bull can urinate freely from the new opening. The bull is ready to use after a 4- to 6-week recovery period.[4–14]

Penile Fixation or Penopexy

Penopexy 1

Penile fixation is a procedure that creates a permanent adhesion between the tunica albuginea of the penis and the ventral body wall, preventing protrusion and intromission. The bull, under GA or heavy sedation, is restrained in right lateral recumbency. The ventral abdomen from the preputial orifice to the scrotum on the left side is prepared for aseptic surgery. Local infiltration with lidocaine along the intended incision line maybe necessary for bulls under heavy sedation.

A 10-cm longitudinal incision is made caudally 2 to 3 cm lateral to the midline and beginning midway between the preputial orifice and the base of the scrotum. Blunt dissection is continued through the subcutaneous connective tissue until the penis is located. The penis is exteriorized through the incision and the dorsal surface is dissected free of all connective tissue, beginning caudal to the reflection of the prepuce and continuing caudally for approximately 10 cm, exposing the tunica albuginea. A corresponding area of the linea alba is likewise prepared and the dorsal surface of the penis and the linea alba are vigorously scarified to provide a tissue bed for adhesions to develop. At this point, it is important to identify the urethral groove on the ventral surface of the penis so that it is not accidentally incorporated in the sutures that will be apposing the two scarified tissue beds. Four to six simple interrupted sutures using nonabsorbable material are preplaced 2 cm apart (**Fig. 10**). Before placing the sutures, care should be taken to ensure the sutures begin caudal to the preputial reflection or fornix and the glans penis is not protruding through the preputial orifice. Each suture should include the dorsal one third of the penis and the linea alba. Subcutaneous sutures are placed with an absorbable material, and the skin is closed with a monofilament nonabsorbable suture. This technique results in a permanent adhesion between the tunica albuginea and the line alba. Ideally, the bull should be rested for 6 weeks, to allow adhesions to develop. Bilateral caudal epididymectomy should be performed in conjunction with this technique.[4–8,10]

Penopexy 2

An alternative technique is to fix the penis to the subcutaneous tissue in the perineal area of the bull. This procedure can be done under mild sedation and caudal epidural anesthesia. The perineal area from the neck of the scrotum to the anus is prepared for aseptic surgery. A 4- to 5-cm skin incision is made over the area of the distal loop of the palpable sigmoid flexure, followed by blunt dissection, to free up and expose the ventral surface of the penis below the attachment of the retractor penis muscle (**Fig. 11**). Two to three simple interrupted sutures or an interrupted horizontal mattress suture using heavy nonabsorbable material are placed in the tunica albuginea laterally on both sides of the penis, avoiding the urethra. It is better to include the distal portion of the retractor penis muscles in the sutures, to help stabilize the penis. The sutures are then passed through the adjacent tough connective tissue found in the perineal area of the bull, and sutured (**Fig. 12**). The skin is then closed with a nonabsorbable suture material. Six weeks are allowed for adhesion formation.[6,12]

Bilateral caudal epididymectomy is also performed in conjunction with this technique.

SUMMARY

The literature contains several other surgical techniques described for teaser bull preparation. Each procedure has its advantages and disadvantages. The procedures discussed in this article are those most familiar to the authors and have worked well in the past. Other techniques reported in the literature include amputation of the penis, preputial pouch formation, creation of a preputial stenosis, and artificial corpus cavernosal thrombosis. All have been attempted at one time or another, but for various reasons they were never favored by the authors. By far the most client-requested technique is PPT. Although the procedure involves extensive surgical and tissue dissection, it is not a complicated surgery. These bulls appear to work well for a number of years. Ultimately, the method elected will be influenced by the owner, veterinarian, field facilities, size of the bull, available help, cost, and open or closed herd.

ACKNOWLEDGMENTS

The illustrations of the surgical procedures were provided by Zeke Proctor.

REFERENCES

1. O'Connor ML. Estrus detection. In: Youngquist RS, Threlfall WR, editors. Current therapy in large animal theriogenology 2. Saunders; 2007. p. 270–8.
2. Smith DR. Estrus detection. In: Morrow DA, editor. Current therapy in theriogenology 2. Saunders; 1986. p. 153–8.
3. Kunkle WE, Sand RS, et al. Effect of body condition on productivity in beef cattle: factors affecting calf crop. In: Fields MJ, Sands RS, editors. CRC Press; 1994. p. 186.
4. Claxton MS. Methods of surgical preparation of teaser bulls. Compendium Contin Educ Pract Vet 1989;11(8):974–81.
5. Wolfe DF. Surgical preparation of estrus-detector males. In: Wolfe DF, Moll HD, editors. Large animal urogenital surgery. Baltimore (MD): Williams and Wilkins; 1998. p. 327–33.
6. Gilbert RO, Fubini SL. Surgical management of specific conditions. In: Fubini SL, Ducharme NG, editors. Farm animal surgery. Saunders; 2004. p. 363–4.
7. Turner AS, McIlwraith CW. Bovine urogenital surgery. Techniques in large animal surgery. 2nd edition. Lea and Febiger; 1989. p. 289–332.
8. Hendrickson DA. Surgical techniques for teaser bull preparation. Techniques in large animal surgery. 3rd edition. Blackwell Publishing; 2007. p. 251–6.
9. Riddell MG. Prevention of intromission by estrus-detector males. In: Wolfe DF, Moll HD, editors. Large animal urogenital surgery. 2nd edition. Baltimore (MD): Williams and Williams; 1998. p. 335–43.
10. Walker DF, Vaughan JT. Bovine and equine urogenital surgery. Philadelphia: Lea and Febiger; 1980. p. 27–36.
11. Morgan G. Surgical correction of abnormalities of the reproductive organs of bulls and preparation of teaser animal. In: Youngquist RS, Threlfall WR, editors. Current therapy in large animal theriogenology 2. Saunders; 2007. p. 243–52.
12. Gill MS. Surgical techniques for preparation of teaser bulls. the veterinary clinics of North America food animal practice. Saunders; 1995. p. 123–35.
13. Belling TH. Preparation of "teaser" bull for use in beef cattle artificial insemination program. J Am Vet Med Assoc 1961;138:670.
14. Noordsy JL. Food animal surgery. 2nd edition. Lenexa (KS): Veterinary Medicine Publishing; 1989. p. 225–8.

Surgery of Obstructive Urolithiasis in Ruminants

Jennifer M. Ewoldt, DVM, MS[a,*], Meredyth L. Jones, DVM, MS[b], Matt D. Miesner, DVM, MS[c]

KEYWORDS

- Urolithiasis • Urethral obstruction • Cystotomy
- Urethrotomy • Cystostomy • Ruminant

The predisposition to obstructive urolithiasis in male ruminants involves a combination of anatomic and dietary factors. Uroliths in male ruminants most frequently lodge in the distal sigmoid flexure, near the insertion of the retractor penis muscle, or in the vermiform appendage (urethral process) of small ruminants.[1] Both of these are areas of narrowed urethral diameter. Urethral obstruction at these sites may result in local rupture of the urethra or urinary bladder rupture.

Struvite (magnesium ammonium phosphate) and apatite (calcium phosphate) uroliths are commonly seen in animals fed high-grain diets,[2,3] whereas animals consuming legumes are predisposed to calcium carbonate uroliths.[4] Silicate stones may be observed in animals grazing silicaceous plants and soils in the western United States and Canada.[5] Calcium oxalate stones may be associated with oxalate-containing plants.[6]

A significant factor in the availability of urolith components and their binding ability is urine pH.[1,2,7] Struvite, apatite, and calcium carbonate uroliths are known to precipitate in alkaline urine.[2,8–10] Struvite crystallization occurs only at a pH range of 7.2 to 8.4, whereas apatite stones develop at a urine pH of 6.5 to 7.5.[11] Urine pH may have little or no effect on silicate or calcium oxalate uroliths.

Total body water balance plays an important role in calculogenesis by its effects on urine volume and concentration, which may be seen in winter and during times of systemic illness, when water consumption is reduced. A negative body water balance contributes to supersaturation of urine, precipitation of crystals, and formation of organic and inorganic crystalloids in urine.

[a] Scott County Animal Hospital, 115 South 16th Street, Eldridge, IA 52748, USA
[b] Department of Clinical Sciences, 111B Mosier Hall, Kansas State University, Manhattan, KS 66506, USA
[c] Department of Clinical Sciences, College of Veterinary Medicine, Kansas State University, 1800 Dennison Avenue, Manhattan, KS 66506, USA
* Corresponding author.
E-mail address: doctorewoldt@aol.com (J.M. Ewoldt).

Vet Clin Food Anim 24 (2008) 455–465
doi:10.1016/j.cvfa.2008.06.003 vetfood.theclinics.com
0749-0720/08/$ – see front matter © 2008 Elsevier Inc. All rights reserved.

Medical treatment of obstructive urolithiasis in ruminants has generally been unrewarding. Some form of surgical intervention is necessary to relieve the obstruction, either by direct removal of the urolith, or by bypassing the obstruction. Some surgical methods result in loss of urinary continence, some end the ability of intact males to breed, and others have many complications, the most common of which is urethral stricture. Cost is always a factor in the treatment of ruminants, many of which are destined for slaughter.

In this article, medical management of urolithiasis is described briefly, followed by surgical management and preventative measures.

EVALUATION AND MEDICAL TREATMENT

Physical examination of animals suspected to have obstructive urolithiasis should include evaluation of the abdominal contour and the underline, which may be altered because of bladder or urethral rupture, respectively. Palpation of the preputial hairs may reveal blood clots, crystals, or small stones. In obstructed small ruminants, the urethra may pulse ventral to the anal sphincter or on digital rectal examination, and abdominal palpation may detect bladder distension or free abdominal fluid. In cattle, rectal palpation may reveal urinary bladder distension. Transabdominal ultrasound may also confirm free abdominal fluid.

The penis should be exteriorized in obstructed small ruminants, which is facilitated by use of sedatives. Acepromazine (0.05–0.1 mg/kg, intravenous or intramuscular)[12,13] and diazepam (0.1 mg/kg, slow intravenous) provide systemic and muscle relaxation. The use of xylazine should be avoided because it promotes diuraesis and may contribute to rupture if the obstruction is not relieved immediately. Alternatively, lumbosacral epidural using 2% lidocaine (1 mL/7 kg) may be used in the place of sedation in small ruminants to relieve discomfort and aid in exteriorization of the penis.

Once the penis is exteriorized, the urethral process of small ruminants may be amputated (see section on surgical treatment). This narrowing of the urethra is a common site of obstruction in these species and may provide temporary relief of the obstruction. The urethral diverticulum at the level of the ischial arch prevents retrograde passage of a urinary catheter into the urinary bladder (**Figs. 1** and **2**).[14–16] Therefore, retrograde catheterization or retropulsion of uroliths is not recommended to avoid further trauma or puncture of the urethra at the level of the diverticulum. Attempts at retropulsion of uroliths may result in overdistention of the urinary bladder as the stone is diverted into the diverticulum, allowing fluid to pass into the bladder, followed by the urolith falling back into the urethra and preventing the bladder from emptying.

Once the obstruction is relieved, treatments to acidify the urine should be initiated in an effort to solubilize additional stones and sediment. Initially, ammonium chloride is administered at a dosage of 200 mg/kg orally, with the dosage adjusted to attain a urine pH of 6.0 to 6.5. Care should be taken in dosing so that systemic overacidification does not occur.

Fluid therapy should be instituted as indicated by the clinical findings and economics of the case. Intravenous fluid therapy will also help stabilize critical patients before surgical treatment, and reduces the risk for anesthetic death due to hyperkalemia-induced arrhythmia. After relief of the obstruction, diuresis is important to replace dehydration, reduce azotemia, and flush the urinary tract. A good choice for intravenous fluid therapy is 0.9% NaCl, although additional electrolyte and acid-base abnormalities should be considered.

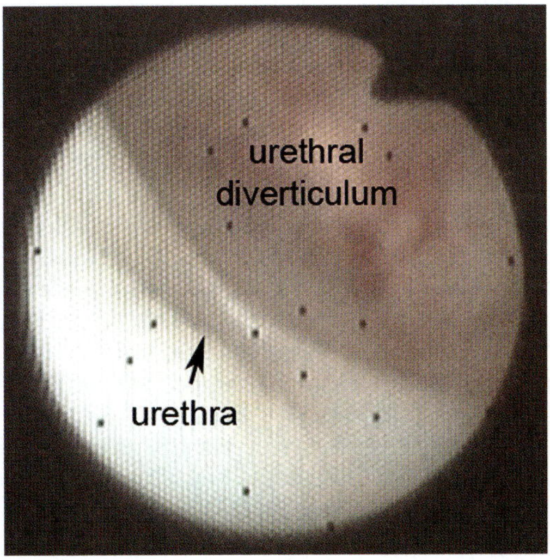

Fig. 1. Endoscopic view of the urethra at the level of the ischial arch. The large cavity to the upper right of the image is the blind pouch of the urethral diverticulum; the narrow opening to the left is the urethra.

Nonsteroidal anti-inflammatory drugs should be administered to decrease inflammation and aid in the prevention of urethral stricture formation, but they should be used with caution until adequate renal perfusion is attained. Broad-spectrum antibiotic therapy should be instituted to prevent or treat infection resulting from devitalized or inflamed urinary tissues, and cavitational accumulation of urine. Beta-lactams (penicillins and cephalosporins) may be chosen because they have a good spectrum of activity and are excreted in the urine.

The goals of medical therapy should include the provision of analgesia, correction of fluid and electrolyte imbalances, treatment or prevention of inflammation or infection, and dissolution of remaining uroliths once the acute obstruction is relieved. Most cases of urethral obstruction will require surgical intervention during the course of case management.

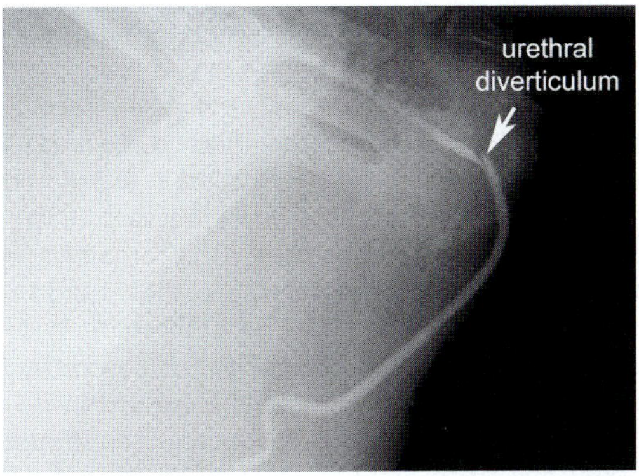

Fig. 2. Contrast urethrogram revealing the urethral diverticulum located at the ischial arch (*arrow*).

SURGICAL TREATMENT

Surgical treatment of urolithiasis in ruminants was traditionally limited to short-term salvage procedures in feedlot animals destined for early slaughter. Success rates varied and depended on the duration of obstruction before surgery, the condition of the animal and the urethral tissue at the time of treatment, concurrent urethral rupture, and the location of the urolith itself. An increase in the number of small ruminants kept as pets has led to the development of new techniques for surgical treatment of urolithiasis. The intent is to develop a corrective procedure that does not stricture rapidly, and does not end the breeding ability of intact males. Research has also led to ways to replace ruptured urethral tissue to salvage animals that would otherwise be doomed to slaughter or euthanasia. The perceived value of these animals as pets also provides the opportunity to perform procedures that would not be cost effective in feedlot animals.

Tube cystostomy for urinary diversion in ruminants was initially described in 1965 as a treatment of ruptured bladders in steers.[17] Since then, it has become popular as a treatment of obstructive urolithiasis in many species of animals, but especially in small ruminants. Rakestraw and colleagues[18] described a case series of 15 small ruminants treated with tube cystostomy, 12 of which were successfully relieved of urinary obstruction. Fortier and colleagues[19] described a group of 25 goats treated with tube cystostomy. A more recent review of 63 small ruminants undergoing tube cystostomy indicated excellent results both short and long term following surgery.[20]

Tube cystostomy provides an alternative surgical treatment to the perineal urethrotomy and urethrostomy techniques previously used to manage urinary obstructions. Long-term outcome of urethrostomy and urethrotomy are reported to be poor.[21,22] Outcome is poor because of stricture formation at the urethrotomy/urethrostomy site, which leads to repeat urethral obstruction.

Urinary diversion techniques, such as antepubic urethrostomy and perineal urethrostomy, are unsuitable for breeding animals because of loss of urethral patency.[21,23] Urinary bladder marsupialization has been described but has been associated with extensive urine scalding problems, stoma stricture, and bladder prolapse through the fistula site.[24,25] Laser lithotripsy, although sometimes used in equine urolithiasis,[26,27] has been described in only a few case reports in ruminants, with some success.[28,29]

The most successful surgical method of treating obstructive urolithiasis in cattle and small ruminants is surgical tube cystostomy.[17,18,20] In this technique, the patient is anesthetized in dorsal recumbency, and the bladder is approached by way of a paramedian incision. A cystotomy is performed to remove any uroliths present, and a Foley catheter (12 to 24 F) is then passed through a stab incision in the body wall of the inguinal region, placed into the bladder through a stab incision, and sutured into place with the cuff inflated (**Fig. 3**). Following closure of the celiotomy incision, an extra catheter is secured with sutures or bandages to the abdominal wall (**Fig. 4**). The catheter is allowed to drain freely for several days, after which it is periodically occluded with a clamp to test for normograde urine flow through the urethra. Once normograde flow is established, the catheter cuff is deflated and the catheter is removed. In two separate reports, urine flow was re-established in a mean of 11.5 and 11 days.[18,20] The success rate of this procedure was 76% to 90% in the short term, and 86% in the long term.[18,20] Success rates have been shown to depend on several factors.[19,20] The major drawback of surgical tube cystostomy is the cost associated with the procedure, because animals must be hospitalized during the waiting period before catheter occlusion. Tube cystostomy has been used to restore breeding function in intact male animals, avoiding the loss of breeding function, as previously described.[30] One of the

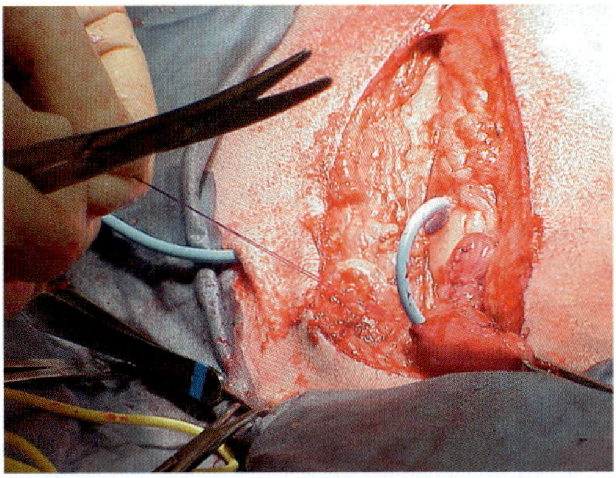

Fig. 3. Intraoperative view of placement of tube cystostomy catheter. The catheter enters the abdomen through the body wall to the left, and is sutured in place in the bladder at the bottom of the image. The sutured cystotomy incision for removal of uroliths can be seen to the right of the catheter.

authors (JME) has experience with this technique in llamas, alpacas, whitetail deer, and a camel, and has anecdotal evidence of its use in potbellied pigs. Success rates vary widely in these alternative species, but the technique is the same.

To reduce the costs associated with the tube cystostomy procedure, a percutaneous tube cystostomy technique has been developed for placement of the cystostomy tube.[31] This technique was successful in the initial description, but subsequent reports indicated that it is 5.6 times more likely to require a second procedure to replace the tube following premature tube loss.[19] If successful, percutaneous tube cystostomy is managed similarly to the surgically placed tubes, in that the tube is periodically occluded after a waiting period of approximately 7 days, and is removed once urination is re-established.

Urinary bladder marsupialization has been moderately successful in restoring urination in goats.[24,25] It does eliminate urinary continence and may, as a result, be

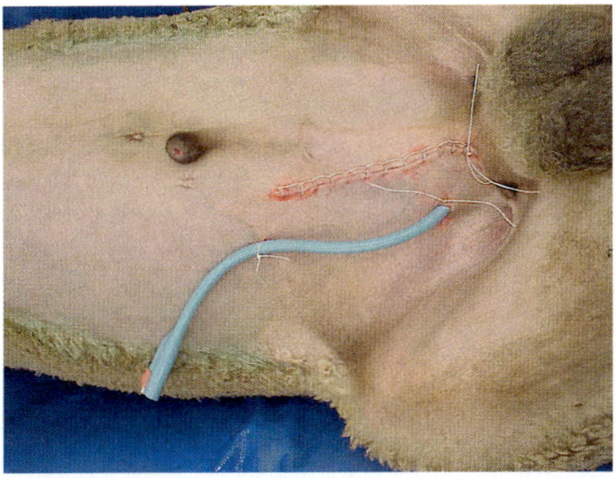

Fig. 4. Completed tube cystostomy procedure, showing the location of abdominal incision and placement of Foley catheter through the abdominal wall. The remaining catheter is sutured to the abdominal wall to keep it elevated and protected.

unacceptable to some pet owners. In this technique, the apex of the bladder is marsupialized to the ventral body wall at midline during a midline celiotomy, creating a stoma that allows for free drainage of urine from the bladder (**Fig. 5**). Major complications include bladder mucosal prolapse through the stoma, urine scald on the ventrum of the animal, and ascending urinary tract infections through the marsupialization site.[24,25] The marsupialization stoma strictured in 3 of 25 goats.[24,25] Success rates were 66% and 94% in two separate studies.[24,25] Hospitalization was significantly shorter than tube cystostomy (mean of 4 days vs. 14 days), which may reduce the cost associated with the procedure.

Prepubic urethrostomy has been described in a sheep and a goat for relief of obstructive urolithiasis.[23] In the report described, prepubic urethrostomy was used for relief of urinary obstruction following perineal urethrostomy stricture formation. The technique used is similar to that performed in dogs and cats. Both animals described were able to void normally after the procedure, but recurrent cystitis and further stricture formation were complications. Because of the proximal location of the surgery in the urethra and the difficulty of the procedure, this technique should be reserved for revision of failed urethroplasties.

Several researchers have recently investigated laser lithotripsy for dissolution of uroliths in ruminants.[28,29] A chromium-thulium-holmium:yttrium-aluminum-garnet (Ho:YAG) laser was used successfully to rupture a urethral calculus when placed through an ischial urethrotomy in a steer, and fractured uroliths in three goats and two potbellied pigs.[28,29] The use of lithotripsy depends on the presence of a urethra sufficiently large for passage of the laser in an endoscope, and positioning of the uroliths in the distal urethra. Lithotripsy, however, presents a viable option for removal of uroliths in the future, and further investigation is warranted. Advantages include reduced cost and rapid discharge from the hospital.

Buccal mucosal grafting has recently been described for the reversal of a perineal urethrostomy in a goat.[32] In this case, the urethra was reconstructed using a strip of tissue from the buccal mucosa following unsuccessful revision of the urethrostomy site. Buccal mucosa proved to be an excellent tissue for this procedure, and healing was excellent, with good long-term survival.

Vesicular irrigation with hemiacidrin was used in conjunction with percutaneous tube cystostomy to restore urinary function in a goat.[31] The investigators concluded that irrigation resulted in rapid dissolution of calcium phosphate uroliths without the

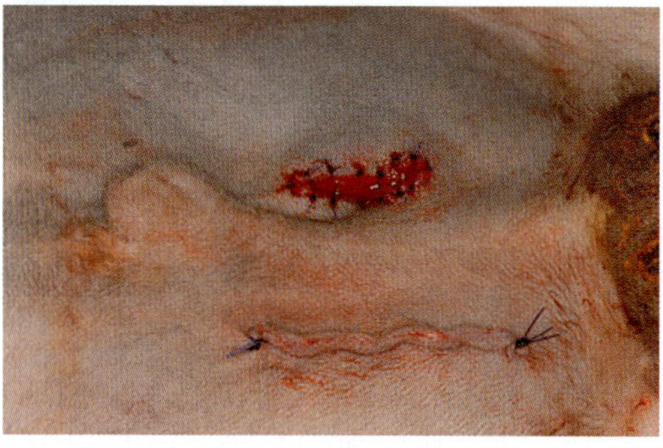

Fig. 5. Completed urinary bladder marsupialization. The stoma is visible at the top of the photo, with the abdominal incision at the bottom of the photo. (*Courtesy of* Kimberly A. May, DVM, MS.)

need for celiotomy and cystotomy. Vesicular irrigation could be combined with surgical or percutaneous tube cystostomy, and perhaps also with other techniques, to dissolve uroliths in situ. The efficacy of this technique on different types of uroliths is not known.

Urolith removal by cystotomy combined with normograde and retrograde urethral flushing was successful in restoring urinary function in seven of eight small ruminants with obstructive urolithiasis.[21] The investigators concluded that this technique was more successful than perineal urethrostomy in restoring urinary function. However, at the time of that study, further techniques such as tube cystostomy, urinary bladder marsupialization, and laser lithotripsy had not been described.

Perineal urethrostomy has long been the mainstay of urolithiasis treatment in ruminants. It is considered a salvage technique in most cases, although some animals have survived for long periods of time after surgery. With this technique, a permanent opening is made in the urethra through which the animal voids urine. Perineal urethrostomy does not guarantee urethral patency because an animal can still obstruct proximal to the stoma. As a result, the urethrostomy stoma should be placed as distal as possible to allow for repeat surgery more proximally if needed. However, the stoma must be located in such a location that it will be proximal to the obstructing urolith. Numerous descriptions of the surgery are available in large animal surgery texts. The technique is usually described as a "high" perineal urethrostomy, located near the ischium, or a "low" perineal urethrostomy, located closer to the scrotum. The most common complication of urethrostomy is stricture of the stoma, which may occur rapidly (weeks to months) after surgery.[33]

Penile amputation (penectomy) is similar to the technique escribed for perineal urethrostomy; however, the penis is transected and may be completely removed rather than creating a stoma in the penis (**Fig. 6**). This procedure is simpler than perineal urethrostomy, but has the disadvantage of increased stricture rate and speed. It is strictly a salvage procedure. Again, the procedure may be performed at a "high" or "low" location, as described in food animal surgery texts.

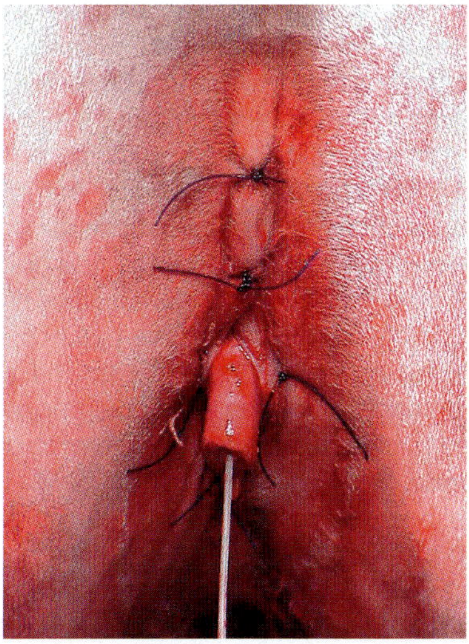

Fig. 6. Perineal urethrostomy with penile transection in a steer. The stay sutures fixating the transected penis are visible, as is a urinary catheter placed in the urethra.

If the urolith is in a location that can be palpated or reached by catheter, a simple urethrotomy can be performed over the urolith itself, or adjacent to the urolith in healthier tissue. Following incision at the urolith, it is removed with forceps or is crushed to allow the pieces to pass. An alternative technique involves retropulsion of a urolith from the distal urethra to an ischial urethrotomy where it can be removed. Urethral stricture formation is a common side effect of urethrotomy, but the simplicity of the procedure makes it popular in breeding animals where the penis must remain intact.[33] The urethrotomy incision may be allowed to heal without suturing because suturing may increase the likelihood of stricture formation. Some surgeons, however, recommend suture closure of the urethrotomy as soon as possible to prevent stricture formation.

PREVENTION

Because of the poor prognosis and expense associated with clinical cases of obstructive urolithiasis and the herd or flock implications of the disease, considerable focus should be placed on prevention. Risk factors to address in preventative strategies include high dietary phosphorus/calcium ratio, high dietary magnesium, low fiber content of rations, low urine output, and an alkaline urine pH. Additional factors, including selective grazing and castration timing, may also be addressed.

Mineral components of uroliths come primarily from the diet, making control of the mineral content of rations particularly important in prevention. In general, phosphorus should never comprise greater than 0.6% of the total ration,[2] and the calcium/phosphorus ratio should be maintained at 2.5:1 or 2:1, achieved by the use of calcium salts, if necessary.[1,3,7,34] High phosphorus levels are present in grains, particularly sorghum, wheat, corn, milo, and oats.[1,10,34] Phosphorus excretion into the urine may be decreased by the feeding of more roughage and the avoidance of pelleted rations, to encourage salivary excretion of phosphorus.[1,2,35] Magnesium control is important even in prevention of uroliths, which do not contain magnesium in their primary structure. It is recommended that magnesium never comprise greater than 0.6% of the total ration[2] and, because the magnesium in roughage diets is less available than that from concentrates,[2] roughage-based diets are preferable.

Increasing water intake and urine volume is an important preventive measure for urolithiasis. Sources recommend the provision of adequate palatable water at desirable temperatures according to the ambient environment[1,2,10,34] and ruminants demonstrate a reduction in water intake for grain feeding over roughage feeding.[2] Water intake is not perfectly tied to urolithiasis because in one study, a decrease of water intake of 20% below normal voluntary intake did not alter the incidence of urolithiasis.[36]

The role of urine pH in urolithiasis is well documented and various sources recommend urine pH goals of 5.5 to 6.5, based on the solubilities of the common stone compositions. Because of an ability to alter acid-base balance and body water balance, salts have been widely used and recommended for the prevention of urolithiasis. Anionic salts containing primarily chlorides have been popular and used extensively because they reduce urine pH, increase urine output, and, ultimately, prevent urolithiasis.[1,2,7,10] Sodium chloride (1%–4%), calcium chloride (1%–2%) and ammonium chloride (0.5%–2%) have been traditionally added to as percentages of rations to increase water intake and produce acidic urine, with inconsistent results.[37–40]

The addition of these salts as a simple percentage of the diet without consideration for the components of the total ration may lead to inconsistent and unsuccessful maintenance of low urinary pH. The concept of dietary cation-anion difference (DCAD) states that with increased cations in the diet, alkalotic tendencies will occur.

Conversely, increased anions in the diet have acidifying potential. Different commercial diets are commonly formulated using various commodities and these commodities are interchanged regularly in feed preparation based on availability. If a feedstuff or a particular batch of feed is higher in cations, or anionic salts are fed in conjunction with high-potassium forage, the DCAD of the diet will be raised and urinary acidification may not occur, despite the addition of the standard dose of anions. This one-dose-fits-all method may be the major cause of sporadic urolith formation in animals being fed anionic salts. The use of DCAD balancing for ruminant urolithiasis is mentioned as a recommendation in some sources,[1,10,41,42] and it is recommended that high cation–containing feedstuffs such alfalfa and molasses be avoided.[10] Few controlled studies for target DCAD levels currently exist, but a DCAD of 0 mEq/kg appears to achieve a urine pH of intact and castrated goats of less than 6.5.[41,42] To assess accurately the efficacy of salts in the diet, whether DCAD balanced or not, owners should be encouraged to assess urine pH periodically at home.

Grazing of female animals on pastures that have high silica content of soil and plants is preferred to the grazing of male animals on these pastures. If male animals are to be grazed in these locations, water intake should be encouraged by maintaining desirable and accessible water sources and supplementation of the anionic salts, ammonium chloride,[43] or sodium chloride,[44] and reduction in the dietary calcium/phosphorus ratio.[44,45]

Early castration is commonly thought to reduce the positive influence of testosterone on urethral diameter and to diminish normal prepucial to penile attachments that are present in the neonate. In calves and in goats, intact animals have shown to have the largest urethral diameters, followed by delayed and partial castrates, with early castrates having the smallest urethral diameters.[46,47] Delaying castration, where production parameters allow, may serve to increase urethral diameter and reduce obstructive rates.

Urolithiasis is multifactorial, making it difficult to design consistently reliable preventative programs. With adherence to the above goals, primarily focusing on dietary modification, significant reductions in clinical cases may be achieved.

SUMMARY

Most cases of obstructive urolithiasis will require surgical intervention at some point during the treatment process. Fluid, anti-inflammatory, antibiotic, and acidifying therapies should be used in support of surgical intervention.

Surgical technique may be chosen based on the characteristics of the individual case, including site of obstruction, location of the rupture, and value of the animal. Prevention remains the mainstay of urolithiasis management. Identification of a case of obstructive urolithiasis should trigger action for the affected individual and the entire herd or flock of origin.

REFERENCES

1. VanMetre DC, Divers TJ. Diseases of the renal system: urolithiasis. In: Smith BP, editor. Large animal internal medicine. 3rd edition. St. Louis (MO): Mosby; 2002. p. 853–60.
2. Hay L. Prevention and treatment of urolithiasis in sheep. Veterinary Record 1991; 12(Suppl):87–91.
3. Hoar DW, Emerick RJ, Embry LB. Potassium, phosphorus and calcium interrelationships influencing feedlot performance and phosphatic urolithiasis in lambs. J Anim Sci 1970;30(4):597–600.

4. Manning RA, Blaney BJ. Epidemiological aspects of urolithiasis in domestic animals in Queensland. Aust Vet J 1986;63:423–4.
5. Bailey CB. Silica metabolism and silica urolithiasis in ruminants: a review. Can J Anim Sci 1981;61:219–35.
6. McIntosh GH. Urolithiasis in animals. Aust Vet J 1978;54:267–71.
7. Jensen R, Mackey D. Urinary calculosis. In: Jensen R, Mackey D, editors. Diseases of feedlot cattle. 3rd edition. Philadelphia: Lea and Febiger; 1979. p. 262–7.
8. Osborne CA, Polzin DJ, Abdullahi SU, et al. Struvite urolithiasis in animals and man: formation, detection and dissolution. Adv Vet Sci Comp Med 1985;29:1–45.
9. Floyd JG Jr. Urolithiasis in food animals. In: Howard JL, Smith RA, editors. Current veterinary therapy 4: food animal practice. Philadelphia: Saunders; 1999. p. 621–4.
10. Pugh DG. Lower urinary tract problems. In: Pugh DG, editor. Sheep and goat medicine. 1st edition. Philadelphia: Saunders; 2002. p. 267–76.
11. Elliot JS, Quaide WL, Sharp RF, et al. Mineralogical studies of urine: the relationship of apatite, brushite and struvite to urinary pH. J Urol 1985;80(4):269–71.
12. Oehme FW, Tillmann H. Diagnosis and treatment of ruminant urolithiasis. J Am Vet Med Assoc 1965;147:1331–9.
13. Van Metre DC, House JK, Smith BP, et al. Obstructive urolithiasis: medical treatment and urethral surgery. Compendium on Continuing Education for the Practicing Veterinarian 1996;18:317–28.
14. Dyce KM, Sack WO, Wensing CJG. The pelvis and reproductive organs of male ruminants. In: Dyce KM, Sack WO, Wensing CJG, editors. Textbook of veterinary anatomy. 3rd edition. Philadelphia: Saunders; 2002. p. 713–22.
15. Garrett PD. Urethral recess in male goats, sheep, cattle, and swine. J Am Vet Med Assoc 1987;220:1831–4.
16. Palmer JL, Dykes NL, Love K, et al. Contrast radiography of the lower urinary tract in the management of obstructive urolithiasis in small ruminants and swine. Vet Radiol Ultrasound 2002;39:175–80.
17. Hastings DH. Retention catheters for treatment of steers with ruptured bladders. J Am Vet Med Assoc 1965;147:1329–30.
18. Rakestraw PC, Fubini SL, Gilbert RO, et al. Tube cystostomy for treatment of obstructive urolithiasis in small ruminants. Vet Surg 1995;24:498–505.
19. Fortier LA, Gregg AJ, Erb HN, et al. Caprine obstructive urolithiasis: requirement for 2nd surgical intervention and mortality after percutaneous tube cystostomy, surgical tube cystostomy, or urinary bladder marsupialization. Vet Surg 2004; 33:661–7.
20. Ewoldt JM, Anderson DE, Miesner MD, et al. Short- and long-term outcome and factors predicting survival following surgical tube cystostomy for treatment of obstructive urolithiasis in small ruminants. Vet Surg 2006;35:417–22.
21. Haven ML, Bowman KF, Englebert TA, et al. Surgical management of urolithiasis in small ruminants. Cornell Vet 1993;83:47–55.
22. Van Weeren PR, Klein WR, Voorhout G. Urolithiasis in small ruminants I. A retrospective evaluation of urethrostomy. Vet Q 1987;9:76–9.
23. Stone WC, Bjorling DE, Trostle SS, et al. Prepubic urethrostomy for relief of urethral obstruction in a sheep and a goat. J Am Vet Med Assoc 1997;210:939–41.
24. May KA, Moll HD, Wallace LM, et al. Urinary bladder marsupialization for treatment of obstructive urolithiasis in male goats. Vet Surg 1998;27:583–8.
25. May KA, Moll HD, Duncan RB, et al. Experimental evaluation of urinary bladder marsupialization in male goats. Vet Surg 2002;31:251–8.
26. Howard RD, Pleasant RS, May KA. Pulsed dye laser lithotripsy for treatment of urolithiasis in two geldings. J Am Vet Med Assoc 1998;212:1600–3.

27. Judy CE, Galuppo LD. Endoscopic-assisted disruption of urinary calculi using a holmium: YAG laser in standing horses. Vet Surg 2002;31:245–50.
28. Streeter RN, Washburn KE, Higbee RG, et al. Laser lithotripsy of a urethral calculus via ischial urethrotomy in a steer. J Am Vet Med Assoc 2001;219:640–3.
29. Halland SK, House JK, George LW. Urethroscopy and laser lithotripsy for the diagnosis and treatment of obstructive urolithiasis in goats and pot-bellied pigs. J Am Vet Med Assoc 2002;220:1831–4.
30. Todhunter P, Baird AN, Wolfe DF. Erection failure as a sequela to obstructive urolithiasis in a male goat. J Am Vet Med Assoc 1996;209:650–2.
31. Streeter RN, Washburn KE, McCauley CT. Percutaneous tube cystostomy and vesicular irrigation for treatment of obstructive urolithiasis in a goat. J Am Vet Med Assoc 2002;221:546–9.
32. Gill MS, Sod GA. Buccal mucosal graft urethroplasty for reversal of a perineal urethrostomy in a goat wether. Vet Surg 2004;33:382–5.
33. Van Metre D. Urolithiasis. In: Fubini SL, Ducharme NG, editors. Farm animal surgery. St. Louis (MO): Saunders; 2004. p. 534–47.
34. Kimberling CV. Diseases of the urinary system: calculosis. In: Kimberling CV, editor. Jensen and Swift's diseases of sheep. 3rd edition. Philadelphia: Lea and Febiger; 1988. p. 205–8.
35. Sockett DC, Knight AP, Fettman MJ, et al. Metabolic changes due to experimentally induced rupture of the bovine urinary bladder. Cornell Vet 1986;76:198–212.
36. Poole DBR. Observations on the role of magnesium and phosphorus in the aetiology of urolithiasis in male sheep. Ir Vet J 1989;43:60–3.
37. Udall RH, Chow FHC. Studies on urolithiasis VII. The effects of sodium, potassium, or chloride ions in the control of urinary calculi. Cornell Vet 1965;55:538–44.
38. Crookshank HR. Effect of ammonium salts on the production of ovine urinary calculi. J Anim Sci 1970;30(6):1002–4.
39. Bushman DH, Embry LB, Emerick RJ. Efficacy of various chlorides and calcium carbonate in the prevention of urinary calculi. J Anim Sci 1967;26:1199–204.
40. Bushman DH, Emerick RJ, Embry LB. Effect of various chlorides and calcium carbonate on calcium, phosphorus, sodium, potassium and chloride balance and their relationship to urinary calculi in lambs. J Anim Sci 1968;27:490–6.
41. Stratton-Phelps M, House JK. Effect of a commercial anion dietary supplement on acid-base balance, urine volume, and urinary ion excretion in male goats fed oat or grass hay diets. Am J Vet Res 2004;65(10):1391–7.
42. Jones M, Streeter RN. Dietary cation anion balancing for the reduction of urine pH in goats. J Vet Intern Med 2005;19(3):412.
43. Stewart SR, Emerick RJ, Pritchard RH. Effects of dietary ammonium chloride and variations in calcium to phosphorus ratio on silica urolithiasis in sheep. J Anim Sci 1991;69(5):2225–9.
44. Bailey CB. Siliceous urinary calculi in calves: prevention by addition of sodium chloride to the diet. Science 1967;155(763):696–7.
45. Stewart SR, Emerick RJ, Pritchard RH. High dietary calcium to phosphorus ratio and alkali-forming potential as factors promoting silica urolithiasis in sheep. J Anim Sci 1990;68(2):498–503.
46. Marsh H, Safford JW. Effect of deferred castration on urethral development in calves. J Am Vet Med Assoc 1957;130:342–6.
47. Kumar R, Kumar A, Singh H, et al. Effect of castration on urethra and accessory sex glands in goats. Indian Vet J 1982;59:304–8.

Umbilical Surgery in Calves

Aubrey N. Baird, DVM, MS

KEYWORDS

• Hernia • Umbilical mass
• Umbilical abscess • Umbilical remnants

Chemical restraint is covered elsewhere and will not be repeated here. Sedation and local anesthesia are adequate and appropriate in the surgical management of umbilical masses in most cases. General anesthesia will take patient movement out of the equation when performing a difficult, complicated surgery, or even a less complicated one that the practitioner is not experienced in performing, thereby reducing postoperative infections resulting from contamination by subcutaneous or umbilical remnant abscesses. However, the author currently uses general anesthesia predominantly for several reasons. First, in his teaching hospital environment, they want the veterinary student to get as much hands-on experience as possible with umbilical surgery, and for their initial experience to be a positive one. Second, their cases may take longer to perform either because of student involvement or because they operate more complicated cases referred from the general practitioner. Calves done with sedation and local anesthesia tend to become restless during prolonged procedures. Finally, they also tend to operate on older, bigger calves, which are more difficult to handle safely without general anesthesia. This situation seems to be the case when umbilical masses develop in the older calf, are first noticed by the owner when the calf is older, or surgical treatment has been delayed for various reasons. However, in a practice situation where time and expense are critical, the author would not hesitate to treat surgically young calves affected by any of the umbilical conditions described in this article with the aid of sedation, local anesthesia, and physical restraint.

INCISION AND CLOSURE

Before surgical preparation and incision, any draining umbilical mass should be sutured closed to prevent contamination of the surgical site. The surgical incision in the heifer is by way of a simple elliptic skin incision around the umbilical mass. Caution should be taken with location of the skin incision to ensure adequate skin remains to allow skin closure without tension. The subcutaneous tissue is dissected around the umbilical mass until the glistening white external sheath of the rectus abdominis

Department of Veterinary Clinical Sciences, School of Veterinary Medicine, Purdue University, Lynn Hall, 625 Harrison Street, West Lafayette, IN 47907-2026, USA
E-mail address: abaird@purdue.edu

Vet Clin Food Anim 24 (2008) 467–477
doi:10.1016/j.cvfa.2008.06.005 **vetfood.theclinics.com**
0749-0720/08/$ – see front matter © 2008 Elsevier Inc. All rights reserved.

muscle is exposed. A small body wall incision (just large enough for the surgeon to insert a finger into the abdominal cavity to palpate for any structures associated with the mass) is made on the midline either cranial or caudal to the mass. The location of the initial incision is based on surgeon preference. When one suspects an abscess of an umbilical remnant caudal or cranial to the mass, it is reasonable to make the initial body wall incision opposite the suspected abscess. Some prefer to make the initial incision lateral to the mass; however, the author is more comfortable with the incision on the midline.[1] Then the surgeon dissects around the hernia sac or mass with an elliptic body wall incision while using fingers or instruments to retract associated structures out of harm's way. The body wall incision can then be continued cranially or caudally as needed because of abscess or involvement of fetal remnants. Most commonly, caudal extension is needed to treat a lesion of the urachus. The midline body wall closure is by the method of surgeon's choice. The author routinely uses #1 vicryl, depending on the animal's size, with a simple continuous pattern after placing one to two near-far-far-near tension sutures. The subcutaneous tissue is closed with absorbable suture in a simple continuous pattern. The skin closure may be done in a simple continuous pattern using nonabsorbable suture to be removed in 10 to 14 days or with absorbable suture if the practitioner or owner so desires. However, most calves that owners wish to have surgically corrected warrant a recheck and suture removal.

The male calf presents more challenge because of the preputial orifice being close to the umbilicus. The elliptic skin incision is only useful when the umbilical mass is less than 3 cm in diameter. For most umbilical masses in male calves, a half-moon or semilunar skin incision is more appropriate. The skin incision is centered over the umbilicus with the concave side directed caudally. Caudal reflection of the sheath is usually adequate to allow an elliptic body wall incision. The semilunar skin incision also allows caudal extension of the skin incision on either side as a paramedian incision. The caudal paramedian skin incision allows reflection of the sheath and prepuce to the contralateral side. The elliptic body wall incision can then be extended as needed. This approach allows access caudally to any urachal abscess or umbilical artery infections without damaging the elastic tissues of the prepuce or the penis itself. The body wall closure is the same as in the female calf. If the skin incision has been extended as a paramedian, the subcutaneous closure is done longitudinally on the line of the paramedian skin incision. Occasional tacking sutures will be helpful to obliterate dead space where the prepuce has been reflected. The subcutaneous closure of the semilunar incision is done transversely. The underline will have a dimple and not be cosmetically pleasing immediately after the surgery. However, the long-term result is acceptable. The skin closure is again surgeon's preference. It is wise to place the first suture at the cranial-most aspect of the semilunar incision and work caudally from that point on each side. This approach makes it much easier to accomplish an even closure.

REMNANTS

Any discussion of umbilical surgery would be remiss in not describing the normal umbilical area and related anatomy (**Fig. 1**). The umbilicus provides circulation and waste disposal in the fetal calf through placental attachment. The paired umbilical arteries are found on either side of the bladder. They carry oxygen-poor blood from the fetus. After birth, these arteries become the lateral ligaments of the bladder. Infection of one or both of the umbilical arteries is called omphaloarteritis. They are normally thick walled with clotted blood inside. Any abscess will be appreciated to be an

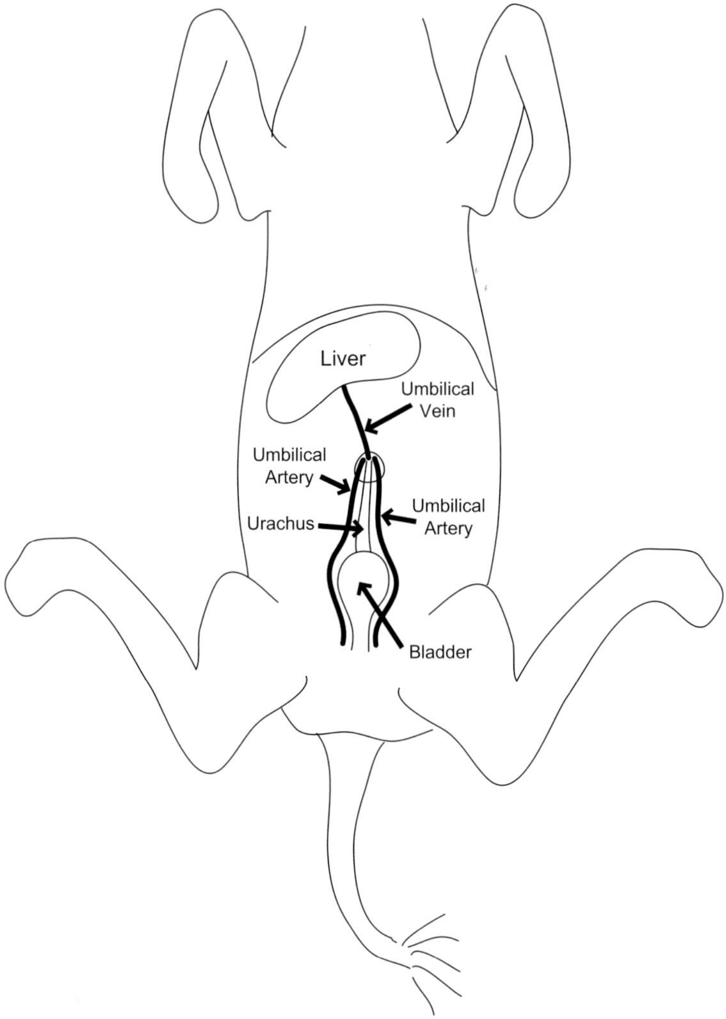

Fig. 1. The normal umbilical remnants in the calf that may become infected and be associated with umbilical masses.

enlargement of the artery, which is otherwise a consistent diameter for the entire length of the structure. The urachus is a fetal continuation of the bladder taking waste to the allantoic sac (**Fig. 2**). It should atrophy shortly after birth and disappear in the normal calf. The umbilical vein courses from the umbilicus cranially into the liver. It delivers oxygen-rich blood and nutrients to the fetus through the liver and ductus venosus. It normally becomes the round ligament of the liver (falciform ligament). Any of these structures can become infected and associated with umbilical masses (**Fig. 3**).[2] Infected umbilical remnants can be associated with an enlarged umbilicus that can be partially reducible or nonreducible; it can be draining purulent exudate frequently or intermittently. Occasionally, an abnormal umbilical remnant is discovered when repairing what is thought to be a simple reducible hernia.

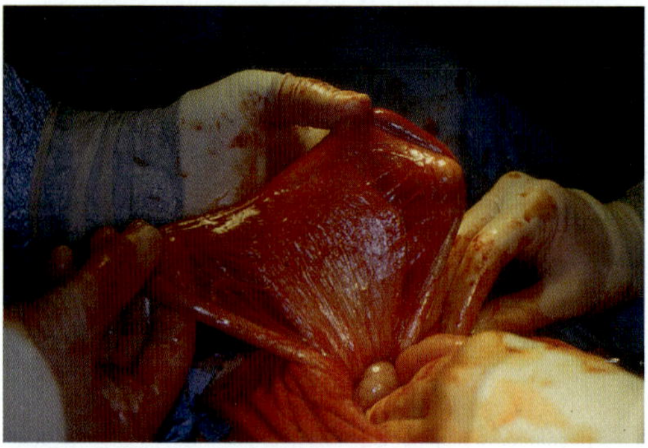

Fig. 2. Intraoperative photograph showing the urachus and bladder with umbilical arteries on either side. (*Courtesy of* Jan Hawkins, DVM, West Lafeyette, IN.)

The tissue making up the normal umbilical cord seen at birth is the urachus and umbilical vein. The umbilical arteries retract into the abdomen as the cord is stretched at birth. Good hygiene is critical at calving to prevent ascending infections of the umbilical cord. It is also frequently difficult to accomplish. Dipping the umbilicus is important, although not easily done in some management situations. Although a calving area that can be closely watched is helpful in some situations, such a confinement area can become a source of infection toward the end of the calving season if strict attention is not paid to cleaning and disinfection. Therefore, calving on clean fresh pasture may be superior to having a calving lot or barn.

EXAMINATION AND CLASSIFICATION

The most important part of the examination of umbilical masses by the practitioner is the manual palpation. First, a size-appropriate restraint should be provided. Young calves can frequently simply be held with one arm around the neck and a hand on the tail. Bigger calves may require two people to accomplish the same restraint. Calves may be placed in lateral recumbency by use of physical restraint alone or combined with a casting rope. The author prefers to use a rope tightened round the

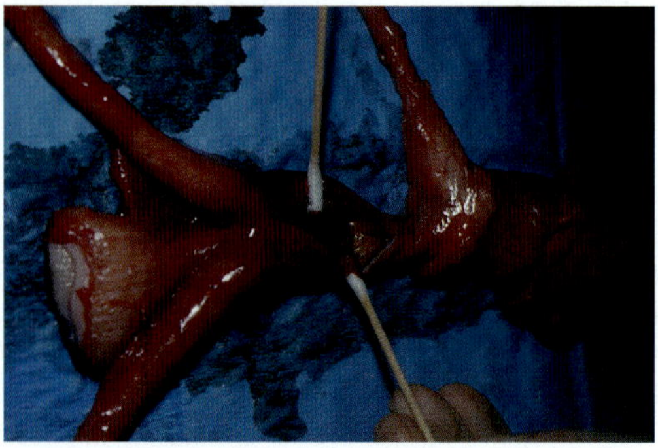

Fig. 3. Surgical specimen with resected umbilical arteries to the left on either side of the resected bladder tip and urachus. The skin is to the right and the umbilical vein is attached in the upper right part of the field. The tips of the cotton swabs are in the opened urachal abscess. (*Courtesy of* Jan Hawkins, DVM, West Lafeyette, IN.)

calf's flank rather than more elaborate patterns required to cast adult cattle. Even larger and more fractious calves may require squeeze chute restraint. The presence of infected umbilical remnants is often easier to determine in the recumbent calf. The author routinely palpates calves while in dorsal recumbency as they are being prepared for surgery. The abdominal relaxation in recumbency allows deeper palpation, which may help identify enlargement of the urachus or umbilical vein within the abdominal cavity. The author has found that the abscessed remnant must still be large to determine its presence reliably on palpation. When the practitioner suspects the presence of a large abscess, he/she can then make the initial body wall opening into the abdominal cavity cranial or caudal to the umbilical mass opposite the enlarged abdominal structure palpated.

The umbilical mass should be palpated to determine if the calf shows any signs of pain when the mass is manipulated. One should thoroughly examine for the presence of any discharge or scab that would indicate previous drainage and then try to reduce the mass while paying particular attention to structures within the mass that may be movable, and reduce into the abdominal cavity. It is helpful if one can identify if the movable contents of the mass are omentum or sections of intestine. Also, one can occasionally palpate adhesions of the hernia contents to the hernia sac. Umbilical masses can be classified as nonreducible, reducible, or partially reducible. If reducible (or partially reducible), the hernia ring should be evaluated for thickness and completeness and the size of the body wall defect should be assessed. A nonreducible mass may indicate an abscess that is either a large cavity full of thick, purulent exudate or multiple foci of infection surrounded by fibrous tissue. One is frequently tempted to simply lance and drain an umbilical abscess. However, that method should be approached with caution because the result could be formation of an abomasal fistula in the case of a Richter's hernia, or alternatively, evisceration or enterotomy in the case of an incorrect diagnosis. Even the best result is often early skin closure and formation of another abscess. One may wish to aspirate the suspected abscess or perform an ultrasound examination.

Ultrasound examination of the umbilicus has been described.[3] Ultrasonography of an umbilical mass may provide good information before surgical resection or an attempt to lance and drain an abscess. Interpretation of ultrasonography of the umbilical remnants can be challenging to the inexperienced clinician. Appropriately interpreted ultrasonography may help the practitioner select which umbilical mass cases they wish to treat surgically in the field. The author does not routinely perform ultrasonography on these cases. He and his colleagues choose to keep the ultrasound machine out of harm's way when performing preoperative examination of the calf and to not spend valuable anesthesia or sedation time when preparing the calf for surgery. Rather, they take the approach that they are prepared to explore the abdomen and treat appropriately whatever lesion is present.

SIMPLE HERNIAS

The case most frequently treated in the field is the simple hernia. This hernia is easily reduced completely and has no associated infected remnants. Classically, simple hernias either contain small intestine (enterocele) or omentum (epiplocele) that is easily replaced in the abdominal cavity by depressing the hernia sac. The contents slide with little to no resistance from the hernia sac into the abdomen. When one releases the sac, the contents return readily. It is important to note the size of the body wall rent when the hernia is reduced. Most simple hernias successfully treated in the field will be no more than 3 fingers in size and have a hernia ring that appears thick and easily palpated. Although the practitioner in the field setting may shy away from performing surgery on calves that have larger hernias, they can certainly be treated successfully. The author frequently has mesh implants available for large hernias, but they are rarely ever used in calves. These calves are held off feed for 24 hours or more to empty the intestinal tract and allow easier apposition of the hernia ring. The bigger hernias are closed with more tension sutures and less often with continuous suture patterns.

The author does suggest only one field surgery of umbilical conditions. When incisional hernias occur or abscesses form, referral is recommended. They can be done in the field, but repeat surgeries often benefit from an experienced surgeon in a hospital setting being able to better debride and resect the abnormal tissue.

OMPHALOPHLEBITIS

Infection of the umbilical vein is easily identified on entering the abdominal cavity. Deep abdominal ligature is usually sufficient to resect the abnormal portion of the umbilical vein completely. In cases where the abnormal vein extends into the liver parenchyma, marsupialization of the vein is indicated.[1,4] This possibility justifies a bigger area of clip and prep than one might think necessary. Marsupialization of the vein can be done at the cranial end of the skin incision and through a separate body wall incision cranial to the skin incision. The author prefers marsupialization through a separate stab incision because it leads to fewer incisional complications. The risk for abdominal contamination is minimal when properly covering the end of the vein during relocation. The separate stab also compliments the semilunar incision described earlier in male calves. The abnormal vein is dissected free at the umbilicus and covered with a surgical sponge and glove to prevent contamination of the abdomen with the contents of the abscess. A circular skin incision is made cranial to the umbilical incision and just to the right of the midline. This positioning allows the vein to exit the abdominal cavity directly ventral to the liver. The size of the circular skin incision is determined by the size of the umbilical vein that will exit the body wall. The external rectus sheath is then either incised in a circular fashion or simply in a linear manner and bluntly enlarged to facilitate the affected vein. The vein is usually sutured with minimal tension to the external rectus sheath with 10 to 12 simple interrupted absorbable sutures. A second layer of suture secures the vein to the skin, again with simple interrupted sutures using nonabsorbable or delayed absorbable material. The vein can be flushed to stimulate drainage and healing but this procedure is not without potential complications. The practitioner should never flush under pressure because the ductus venosus could become patent and allow flush solution and infection to enter the systemic circulation.[4] Certainly, the calf should receive systemic antibiotics during the postoperative period. Frequently, establishing ventral drainage is all that is needed to allow the infection of the vein to resolve. Owners should be informed that a second surgery may be required after the infection has resolved, to resect the vein and close the defect in the body wall. However, the author has found that few of the calves that have a marsupialization have required the second surgery. The healed vein usually atrophies and the defect in the body wall seals over nicely. One is justified in being concerned about the band of umbilical vein leading to entrapment of intestine, such as has been reported with other umbilical remnants.[5,6] However, the author has never seen this complication or any such report in the literature.

URACHUS

The more commonly infected umbilical remnant is the urachus (**Fig. 4**). The calf is less likely to have a patent urachus draining urine like some other large animal species. Any

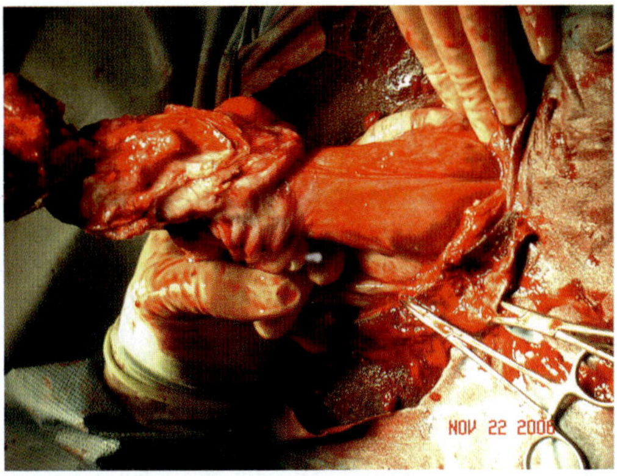

Fig. 4. Surgical photograph of an urachal abscess. The surgeon's left hand holds the umbilical vein and adhered omentum. The incised skin is to the left of the field and the abscessed urachus exits the abdominal incision from the right. (*Courtesy of* Jan Hawkins, DVM, West Lafeyette, IN.)

abnormal urachus in the calf is nearly always an abscess, although urachal cysts have been reported in calves which present with nonreducible, fluctuate umbilical mass.[7] The calf may have an umbilical mass that periodically drains purulent exudate with minimal abscess within the abdominal cavity. Alternatively, the mass outside the body wall may be small and the abscess inside the abdominal cavity may be much larger than the calf's urinary bladder. Some calves may present with pollakiuria. The frequent urination of small volumes is related to the urachal remnant not allowing the bladder to fully decompress and therefore the animal has the frequent urge to urinate. One can occasionally determine the presence of an urachal abscess in young calves by deep transabdominal palpation. This palpation becomes more difficult as the calf grows larger. It is easier to palpate bigger calves in dorsal recumbency while sedated or under general anesthesia. Ultrasound examination is discussed in this article. The author does not routinely use ultrasonography for the calf umbilicus. He and his colleagues take the approach that the animal needs surgery and they will correct the problems they find at surgery. However, it could be argued that ultrasonography could be helpful in determining which cases might be too involved for the practitioner to operate with sedation and local anesthesia only in a field setting. As for the surgical excision of the urachal abscess, the skin and body wall incision is made as described earlier. One must continue the body wall incision caudally to allow the apex of the bladder to be exteriorized. The author packs off the apex of the bladder and attached urachus with moist towels. The urachus and tip of the bladder should be resected. Leaving a portion of the urachus may lead to a urachal diverticulum that does not empty completely at urination and therefore could contribute to cystitis. The author places stay sutures using 0 monofilament suture on either side of the bladder near the apex. The tip of the bladder and urachus are sharply resected near the apex. Suction is used to remove the urine from the bladder. In the absence of suction, one could aspirate the urine using a large syringe. Some surgeons prefer placing doyen forceps across the bladder rather than stay sutures. Again, different surgeons prefer different methods of bladder closure. The author uses 0 or 2-0 Vicryl to close the mucosa in a simple continuous pattern, making every effort not to penetrate the mucosa. He then closes the seromuscular layer with an inverting pattern, such as Cushing or Lembert, with the same suture material. This closure should achieve a fluid-tight seal that does not leak urine.

Another urachal condition involves uroperitoneum in older cattle (frequently yearlings) due to a perforation in a persistent urachus. The owner usually has not noticed any abnormal signs in these animals before the abdominal distention caused by its filling with urine. The animal that has uroperitoneum will develop azotemia and uremia. Rectal palpation of these animals usually reveals an elongated, cylindric bladder, the apex of which the clinician cannot reach around. Extremely sick animals may be treated by draining the abdominal fluid while administering intravenous fluids. One should be careful not to remove abdominal fluid too rapidly without giving intravenous fluids because the rapid fluid shift may lead to collapse of the animal. The author treats these animals by way of a standing left flank laparotomy. On incision into the abdominal cavity, urine dorsal to the ventral aspect of the incision will obviously pour from the abdomen. The author and his colleagues purposefully do not drain any more urine from the abdomen. The urachal remnant will be attached to the ventral abdomen at the umbilicus. One can grasp the urachal remnant, usually wrapping it around one's hand and wrist to better apply traction, and bluntly detach it from the body wall. Frequently, the amount of fibrin associated with the urachus and abdominal floor is considerable. Exteriorizing the urachus and bladder apex through the flank incision will reveal rents in the urachus. The tip of the bladder is exteriorized at the incision site with relative ease. The urachus can then be resected and the bladder closed as described in the calf that has a urachal abscess. Before closing the flank incision, a stab incision is made in the flank through which an equine nasogastric tube is placed into the abdominal cavity extending to the ventral abdomen. The tube is sutured in place and a one-way valve is placed on the end of the tube. This valve can be a commercially available valve or one may simply cut the finger tip out of a surgical glove and tape the glove to the external end of the tube. The tube allows the urine to slowly exit the abdominal cavity over a period of 3 to 5 days. Therefore, the animal may not need intravenous fluids to prevent a catastrophic fluid shift associated with rapid drainage of the abdominal urine.

UMBILICAL ABSCESS

Older calves frequently present with a nonreducible umbilical mass. It can either be in the form of a thickened umbilical cord or a bigger ovoid mass. It is usually not painful to palpation. It may be draining purulent exudate or have signs of previous drainage, such as a scar or scab. Alternatively, no signs may exist of any break in the skin at all. This abnormality is not associated with a body wall defect or intra-abdominal infections of the umbilical remnants. It is truly an umbilical abscess. Calves tend to wall these off nicely and seldom show any clinical signs. Occasionally, a calf that has a large abscess will be unthrifty. Those described as a thickened cord usually contain several small areas of abscess surrounded by fibrous tissue. Often, these abscesses become less noticeable as the calf grows. The true umbilical abscesses may be treated by opening the abscess to drain. However, one should be careful to be sure the calf actually has an abscess. Aspiration with a needle and syringe should be done before opening the abscess. The purulent exudate present in the umbilical abscess will usually be thick. Therefore, one must use a 16- or 14-gauge needle to aspirate because smaller needles seldom yield positive results. Long-term results may be better when these abscesses are treated with surgical resection rather than drainage because opening the abscess to drain will still require repeated flushing to achieve proper healing and to prevent the abscess from resealing when still containing a nidus of infection.

OTHER CONDITIONS

A Richter's (or parietal) hernia may also be mistaken for an abscess by the most experienced of practitioners. The Richter's hernia contains one wall of a luminal organ in the hernia. These hernias are often associated with an intense inflammatory reaction and frequently edema. The calf will not show signs of intestinal obstruction; the normal flow of ingesta continues because only one wall of the intestine is entrapped in the hernia. The most frequent section of intestine entrapped in the Richter's hernia in calves is the abomasum. As such, if one mistakes the Richter's hernia for an umbilical abscess and treats by establishing drainage, one will, in fact, create an abomasal fistula. Occasionally, a fistula will form without intervention.[8] The calf that has an abomasal fistula draining ingesta will develop electrolyte abnormalities that will then complicate anesthesia to repair the fistula. If such a fistula occurs, the surgical treatment of choice is to make an elliptic incision and perform an en bloc resection of the fistula.[9] The practitioner should close the abomasum as any luminal organ and close the body wall. Fistula repair in adult cattle after an abomasopexy technique has been described using wire tension sutures through the entire body wall, with stents. This technique is used because of tension on the closure and contamination of the surgical site. That specific repair is beyond the scope of this discussion on calf umbilical surgery. The calf that has this fistula is nearly always a candidate for primary closure as described for standard umbilical surgery in this article.

Another umbilical abnormality rarely seen at birth is an omphalocele. An omphalocele occurs when one of the four body folds fails to migrate normally in embryologic development. This condition is described as having the appearance of a hernia covered by a paper-thin membrane (amnion) rather than hair. One can usually appreciate the presence of small intestine in the hernia, and sometimes a portion of the liver. If the cow is allowed to clean the calf without human intervention, she may actually rupture the amnion and cause an open hernia with intestine exposed to the environment (**Fig. 5**). This condition has been reported in kittens, humans, and calves.[10] In humans, it is frequently associated with other congenital anomalies, especially ones affecting the heart. Other congenital anomalies have not been described in veterinary reports. These cases usually present as newborn calves because of owner concern about the "hairless hernia" or because the amnion has ruptured, causing an open hernia. However, the author has treated one calf that had grown to be 400 pounds before the open hernia developed and the owner sought veterinary care for the calf. The treatment of

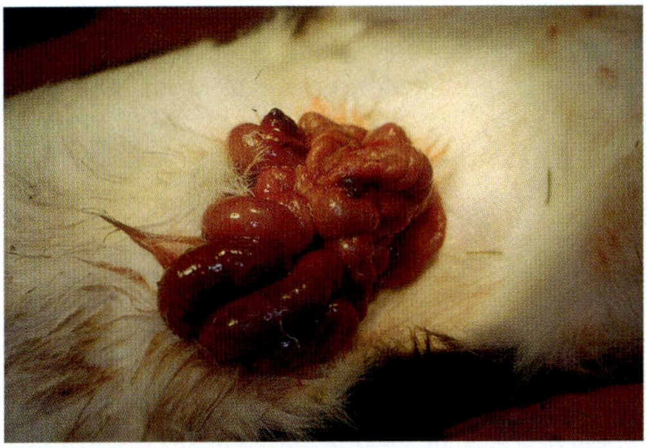

Fig. 5. Open hernia after amnion rupture in an omphalocele. (*Courtesy of* Jan Hawkins, DVM, West Lafeyette, IN.)

this condition is obviously herniorrhaphy. More important than the ultimate treatment is the initial first aid delivered by the attendant who first sees the affected calf. If the tissue covering the hernia is still intact, reduction of the hernia and placement of an abdominal bandage before immediate transport to a veterinarian or calling a practitioner to the farm is the first aid treatment of choice. This procedure can certainly be a field procedure because the newborn calf is small enough to restrain safely in dorsal recumbency and a line block is adequate anesthesia. Another calf that had an omphalocele treated by the author arrived at his clinic before 6 hours of age. The calving was attended and unassisted. The owner consulted the author and his colleagues immediately when he discovered the abnormal umbilicus. Before he returned to bandage the calf, as instructed, the hernia became open as the cow was aggressively cleaning the calf. When the calf arrived at the clinic, she was held in dorsal recumbency on the floor. The herniated small intestine was not reducible through the defect in the body wall. The intestine was congested, desiccated, and grossly contaminated. The body wall defect was elongated cranially after minimal clipping, prep, and infusion with local anesthetic. The intestine was cleaned quickly and placed in a sterile palpation sleeve. The sleeve containing the intestine was placed into the abdominal cavity and the skin and body wall were closed as one layer with continuous suture. The ventral abdomen was then clipped and prepped appropriately for surgery. The sutures used to close the abdomen were then removed. The incision was slightly elongated to allow easy retrieval of the palpation sleeve and previously herniated intestine. The condition of the intestine improved while in the abdominal cavity and was determined to be viable. The intestine was thoroughly cleaned and returned to the abdomen. Carboxymethylcellulose was placed in the abdominal cavity to decrease adhesion formation efore the incision was closed routinely. The calf was treated with antibiotics and anti-inflammatories. She had a low-grade fever but was doing well enough clinically to be discharged from the hospital 4 days after surgery. She developed an incisional hernia that was repaired at 2 months of age. A limited exploration of the abdominal cavity at that time revealed no adhesions or other abnormalities. The heifer went on to show well at the regional level and is currently being used as a brood cow.

SUMMARY

Calves benefiting from umbilical surgery can be affected by several different conditions. However, the practitioner should be able to correct any of these conditions surgically, especially in young calves, as a field procedure. Like other aspects of veterinary practice, the individual must decide what services he/she wishes to offer clients in the field or clinic setting and which ones will be referred. The objective of this article is to equip practitioners who wish to treat umbilical masses surgically with the information they need.

ACKNOWLEDGMENTS

The artwork for **Fig. 1** was provided by Mal Hoover.

REFERENCES

1. Trent AM, Smith DF. Surgical management of umbilical masses with associated umbilical remnant infections in calves. J Am Vet Med Assoc 1984;185(12):1531–4.

2. Baxter GM. Umbilical masses in calves: diagnosis, treatment, and complications. Compendium on Continuing Education for the Practicing Veterinarian 1989;11(4):505–13.
3. Watson E, Mahaffey MB, Crowell W, et al. Ultrasonography of the umbilical structures in clinically normal calves. Am J Vet Res 1994;55(6):773–80.
4. Steiner A, Christoph JL, Oertle C. Marsupialization of umbilical abscesses with involvement of the liver in 13 calves. Vet Surg 1993;22(3):184–9.
5. Hylton WE, Rousseaux CG. Intestinal strangulation associated with omphaloarteritis in a calf. J Am Vet Med Assoc 1985;186(10):1099.
6. Baxter GM, Darien BJ, Wallace CE. Persistent urachal remnant causing intestinal strangulation in a cow. J Am Vet Med Assoc 1987;191(5):555–8.
7. Lischer CJ, Iselin U, Steiner A. Ultrasonographic diagnosis of urachal cyst in three calves. J Am Vet Med Assoc 1994;204(11):1801–4.
8. Fubini SL, Smith DF. Umbilical hernia with abomasal-umbilical fistula in a calf. J Am Vet Med Assoc 1984;184(12):1510–1.
9. Field JR. Umbilical hernia with abomasal incarceration in a calf. J Am Vet Med Assoc 1988;192(5):665–6.
10. Baird AN. Omphalocele in two calves. J Am Vet Med Assoc 1993;202(9):1481–2.

Surgery of the Bovine Large Intestine

Mireille Meylan, Dr med vet, FVH, MS, PhD, Dr habil

KEYWORDS

- Cecal dilation • Atresia • Colon • Malformation
- Field surgery • Cattle

This article consists of a short review of the anatomy of the bovine large intestine, and a more thorough description of the two most relevant diseases of the large intestine amenable to field surgery: cecal dilatation and dislocation (CDD) in cows and intestinal atresia in calves. Rectal prolapse is addressed in another article in this issue.

In disorders affecting the large intestine, as in any other disease, a complete history and careful physical examination are prerequisites for successful treatment, which includes not only surgical intervention but also pre- and postoperative medical treatment. The clinical examination of cattle that have abdominal disease has been described in detail.[1–3]

ANATOMY OF THE BOVINE LARGE INTESTINE

The bovine large intestine consists of the cecum, the ascending, transverse, and descending colon, and the rectum (**Fig. 1**). The cecum usually lies in the supraomental recess with its blind end directed caudally toward the pelvis. It is connected ventrally to the ileum by the ileocecal fold, which contains blood vessels and nerves, and dorsally to the proximal loop of the ascending colon (PLAC) through the short cecocolic band. At the ileocecocolic junction, the cecum continues as the PLAC without visible transition. After extending cranially to the level of the 12th rib, the PLAC turns back laterally until it reaches the caudal flexure of the duodenum. There, it turns around cranially and continues as the spiral colon (spiral loop of the ascending colon), which is embedded in its mesentery in the form of a flat oval. The spiral colon consists of centripetal and centrifugal coils (with 1.5 to 2 revolutions each). The distal loop of the ascending colon runs first in a caudal, then in a cranial direction, and leads to the descending colon over the short transverse colon, which crosses from the right to the left side of the abdomen in front of the cranial mesenteric artery. The rectum lies mostly in the peritoneal part of the pelvic cavity.[4–7]

Clinic for Ruminants, Vetsuisse Faculty of the University of Berne, Bremgartenstrasse 109A, 3012 Berne, Switzerland
E-mail address: mireille.meylan@knp.unibe.ch

Vet Clin Food Anim 24 (2008) 479–496
doi:10.1016/j.cvfa.2008.06.002 **vetfood.theclinics.com**
0749-0720/08/$ – see front matter © 2008 Elsevier Inc. All rights reserved.

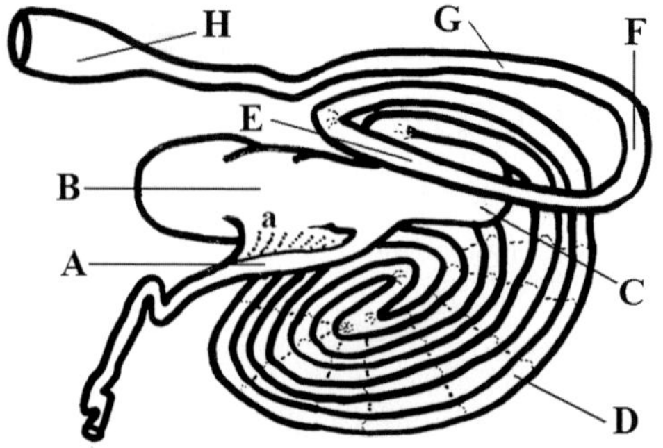

Fig. 1. The bovine large intestine. A, ileum; B, cecum; C, proximal loop of the ascending colon; D, spiral loop of the ascending colon; E, distal loop of the ascending colon; F, transverse colon; G, descending colon; H, rectum; a, ileocecal fold. The cecocolic fold between the cecum and the proximal loop of the ascending colon is not visible under the distal loop of the ascending colon.

CECAL DILATATION AND DISLOCATION

Clinical Presentation and Diagnosis

CDD is a common and economically important abdominal disorder that affects mainly dairy cattle. In an epidemiologic study in Switzerland, similar prevalences (0.05% at individual cow level) were found for CDD and abomasal displacement.[8] The pathologic features of the condition include distention, displacement, and, in some cases, retroflexion or torsion of the cecum and proximal portion of the colon, leading to partial or complete obstruction of the passage of digesta. A retroflexion of the cecum is defined as a displacement of the cecal apex from its normal position toward the pelvic inlet in a cranial direction. A cecal torsion is present if a twist of the cecum occurs along its longitudinal axis, leading to increased tension on the ileocecal fold, thus jeopardizing blood circulation and innervation of the organ. Cecal torsion occurs less frequently than CDD with or without retroflexion.[7]

The clinical presentation of the disease has been described in numerous clinical reports.[3,7,9–16] Typical clinical signs include acute onset of mild colic, a normal to moderately elevated heart rate, decreased appetite, reduced rumen motility, decreased to absent fecal output, distention of the right flank, and positive succussion and percussion auscultation of the right flank (in the dorsal part of the paralumbar fossa, over an area extending caudally to the tuber coxae). In a retrospective study of 111 cases, rectal examination was considered the most reliable diagnostic investigation for CDD, with swinging and percussion auscultation of the right flank.[16] In that report, the distended, displaced, or twisted cecum could be palpated at rectal examination in 95% of the affected animals. In the case of a simple dilatation, the cecal apex is easily recognizable as a rounded, dome-shaped structure, with a diameter of approximately 15 cm, extending into the pelvic inlet. If a retroflexion is present, the body of the cecum, but not the apex, can be palpated as a large, rounded, tense structure in front of the pelvis; rectal palpation alone does not always allow for differentiation of cecal dilatation with retroflexion from right abomasal displacement or volvulus. Cecal torsion can often be identified on rectal examination: in addition to the typical dilated cecal apex, the ileocecal fold is palpable as a taut, twisted, and painful band. Dilated loops of small intestine and of the spiral colon are often encountered on rectal examination of animals that have CDD.[15–17] The appearance of the dilated cecum at ultrasonography from the right flank has been described.[18,19] Blood chemistry values and acid-base status are mostly normal in cows that have CDD. Changes similar to those seen with obstruction of the small intestine (hypokalemic, hypochloremic metabolic alkalosis) can be seen in protracted cases, or if retroflexion or torsion of the cecum is present.[15,20] In one study, hypocalcemia was observed in 48% of 79 affected animals.[20] In the same study, elevated packed cell volume values indicating circulatory compromise were present in only 13% of 86 patients. The concentration of chloride ions in rumen fluid was normal (<25 mmol/L) in 83% of 93 animals that had CDD, whereas it was elevated in the remaining 17%.[20]

Although an association between the occurrence of CDD and season, age of the animals, stage of pregnancy, or time after parturition has not been demonstrated, some investigators report a trend to more frequent occurrence of the disease during the fall and winter months.[11,14–16]

The main differential diagnoses for CDD include right displacement of the abomasum or abomasal volvulus, small intestinal ileus, complete or partial volvulus of the mesentery, or other causes of abdominal pain (eg, pyelonephritis).[11,16,21]

Etiopathogenesis

Despite numerous clinical descriptions of CDD, the pathogenesis of the disease remains poorly understood. In the past, atony or dysmotility of the cecum and PLAC, leading to accumulation of gas and digesta, and followed by dilatation and secondary displacement of the cecum, has been hypothesized to be of primary relevance in the pathogenesis of CDD.[11,12,21,22] However, the patterns of myoelectric activity observed in the cecum and PLAC of cows that showed delayed recovery or recurrence of CDD after surgical correction presented a striking similarity to those recorded immediately orad to a mechanical obstruction in the distal PLAC of an experimental cow. These observations led to the hypothesis that decreased motility preventing normal transit of ingesta might be present not in the cecum itself but in the spiral colon.[23,24]

Alterations in mRNA expression of receptors involved in the regulation of gastrointestinal motility, such as adrenergic,[25] serotonergic,[26] and muscarinic[27] receptors, have been reported in the ileum and large intestine, especially the spiral colon, of cows that have CDD, but it remained unclear whether the observed changes indicate that these receptors are involved in the pathogenesis of the disease or if they are a bare consequence of cecal dilatation.

Elevated concentrations of volatile fatty acids (VFA) in intestinal contents, as observed in cattle fed carbohydrate-rich diets, have been suspected of inhibiting gastrointestinal motility. Total VFA concentrations similar to those in the rumen have been reported for the bovine large intestine.[22,28] Cecal-colonic fermentation accounts for 8.6% to 16.8% of total VFA production in sheep,[29] and the efficiency of the large intestine for VFA production is similar to that of the rumen.[30] Starch resistant to microbial digestion in the rumen (bypass starch) is partially digested enzymatically in the small intestine and partially fermented in the large intestine, the rest being excreted in the feces. Corn starch, especially, is fermented much more slowly than starch from other cereals, thus resulting in large proportions of bypass starch and increased postruminal fermentation.[22,30] When increased amounts of fermentable carbohydrates reach the large intestine, more VFA are produced there by microbial fermentation.[30,31] Several investigators have reported the effects of increased VFA concentrations or high-concentrate diets on ruminant gastrointestinal motility. However, their results are contradictory, with five studies[22,32–35] reporting inhibition of motility with increased VFA levels and three investigators[36–38] being unable to detect an effect on motility parameters. Nevertheless, VFA concentrations were found to be elevated in the contents of cecum, PLAC, and rectum in cows that had spontaneous CDD, as compared with healthy control cows, but it remained unclear if this elevation of VFA was the cause or the consequence of reduced motility and stasis of digesta.[39] In contrast, comparison of the contractility of ex-vivo intestinal wall specimens from the cecum and spiral colon of healthy cows with or without preincubation with VFA did not reveal significant differences.[40] An abrupt increase of concentrates in the diet of healthy dairy cows (from 0% to 50% of the ration over 60 hours) did cause a significant increase of VFA concentrations in large intestinal ingesta, but no relevant inhibition of the myoelectric activity of the spiral colon was observed.[41] In conclusion, elevated VFA concentrations do not appear to play a predominant role in the regulation of bovine intestinal motility or in the pathogenesis of CDD.

Several cows with CDD have been referred to the author's clinic for treatment during outbreaks occurring in herds after introduction of rumen buffers, but these cases could not be documented in detail and a possible role of rumen buffers in the pathogenesis of CDD remains speculative.

Therapy of Cecal Dilatation/Dislocation

Various approaches to the treatment of CDD have been reported. According to earlier reports, attempts at conservative therapy of CDD were first considered useless or even contraindicated.[10,11,21] It is now accepted that in the early stages of the disease, when the general condition of the affected animal remains good, when some feces are still passed, and in cases where a torsion or retroflexion of the cecum can be ruled out by physical examination, conservative treatment with prokinetic drugs, purgatives, or intravenous infusions may be attempted.[14,42] Administration of neostigmine (87.5 mg in 5 or 10 L of isotonic saline solution supplemented with 5% dextrose as a continuous intravenous infusion at a rate of 1–2 drops per second)[42,43] or of bethanechol (0.07 mg/kg subcutaneously, every 8 hours for 2 days)[44] have been advocated. Paraffin oil (3 L) or sodium sulfate (300 g in 10 L water) administered per stomach tube have been described as adequate purgatives for conservative or postoperative treatment of CDD.[14,42]

In more advanced cases, if no improvement occurs on medical treatment, or when a retroflexion or torsion of the organ is suspected, surgical correction of the condition by means of a right flank laparotomy, allowing drainage of the cecum and PLAC contents, is the therapy of choice (see Refs.[7,11,13,15,21,42]). The intervention is best performed under local anesthesia of the right flank (eg, using a proximal or distal paravertebral block) with the animal standing. Positioning the animal in left recumbency with or without general anesthesia, while preventing the risk of the patient lying down during surgery, renders manipulation of the dilated intestine more difficult because the weight of the filled cecum pulls it away from the incision to the left (down) side of the abdomen. After surgical preparation and local anesthesia, a 25- to 30-cm incision is made either vertically in the middle of the right paralumbar fossa or slightly more caudally in a caudodorsal to cranioventral direction. The abdomen is opened in a routine manner. After exploration of the abdominal cavity, an additional plastic drape is added to minimize contamination of the sterile draping around the incision, and the apex of the cecum is exteriorized (**Fig. 2**), which is best achieved by gently pushing the cecum from behind toward the body wall with the palm of the hand. Grasping the cecal wall and pulling toward the incision should be avoided because it bears an increased risk for rupture of the distended cecum. The apex is fixed on both sides by the assistant surgeon with two sterile gauzes, incised over approximately 4 cm, and the contents of the cecum are drained. The ingesta in the exteriorized part of the cecum normally flow freely out of the incision (unless

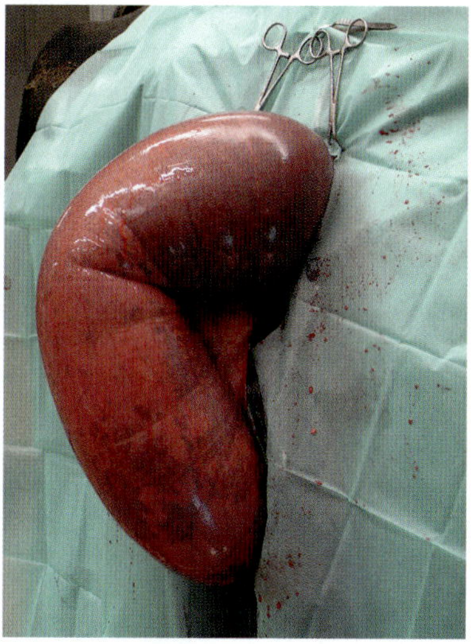

Fig. 2. The dilated cecum is exteriorized through a right flank incision for drainage of its contents.

they are especially dry) and additional material is massaged outside of the abdominal cavity from the rest of the cecal body and the PLAC (**Fig. 3**). When no additional material can be removed, the incision is closed with an inverting pattern (Cushing or Lembert) using absorbable material (eg, 2-0 polyglyconate or polyglactin 910). The cecal apex is copiously flushed with warm saline solution and replaced in the abdomen. In some cases, intestinal contents flow into the cecum from the distal small intestine or from the colon after reposition. If the cecum fills again with a large volume of ingesta, the apex is exteriorized and the suture is reopened to allow for further

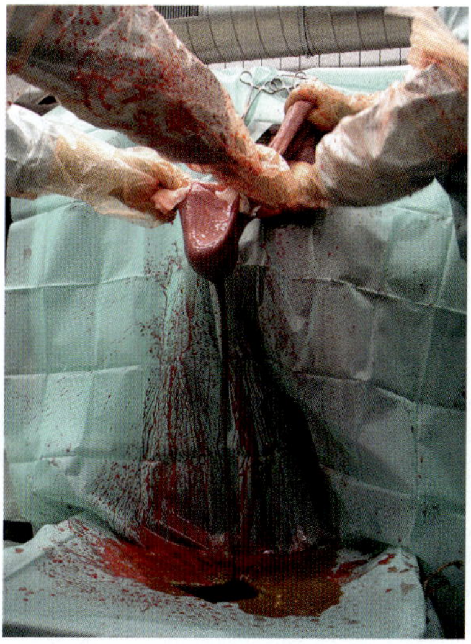

Fig. 3. A stab incision of the cecal apex allows for drainage of its contents. Contents from the cecal body and from the PLAC are massaged in the direction of the cecal apex.

removal of cecal contents. It may be necessary to repeat this procedure several times, but usually not more than once or twice. Contents of the spiral colon often do not flow back into the cecum and are eliminated as feces when large intestinal motility returns after decompression of the cecum. When the cecum remains empty after reposition in the abdomen, a second layer of suture is added using the same pattern to close the cecal apex definitively (**Fig. 4**). After extensive flushing, the cecum is repositioned in the abdomen in its normal anatomic position with the apex directed caudally. The abdominal cavity is closed routinely.[45]

Postoperative care includes antibiotics for 5 days (eg, 30'000 IU Na-penicillin intravenously three times a day), anti-inflammatory drugs as needed (eg, flunixin meglumine, 2 mg/kg intravenously once daily for 1 or 2 days), and infusions of saline or polyionic solutions according to the results of blood chemistry analysis or to the expected changes (hypochloremia, hypokalemia, alkalosis). Under field conditions, the use of a penicillin product with depot effect (eg, procaine penicillin) requiring only one daily application may be preferred, and fluid replacement can be performed through drenching of 20 to 30 L of salt solution into the rumen. Restrictive feeding as part of the therapy for CDD has been described.[14,42] At the author's clinic, no feed is offered on the day of surgery for correction of CDD (day 1), 25% of the calculated ration is offered on the second day, 75% on the third day, and 100% from the fourth day onwards. The animals should be monitored clinically for signs of recurrence for several days after surgery, with normalization of fecal output and rumen activity together with the absence of dilated intestines at rectal palpation indicating normal recovery from CDD.[14,42]

Partial typhlectomy is recommended if the cecal wall is devitalized (eg, after cecal torsion) or if CDD recurs after a first surgical intervention.[7,12,15,43] In such cases, drainage of cecal contents is performed as described earlier, but when the cecum is empty, it is exteriorized as far as possible through the flank incision and an amputation is performed. First, the ileocecal fold is infiltrated with 2% lidocaine to minimize pain at manipulation and thus the risk of the animal trying to lie down. Mass ligatures (eg, with overlapping simple interrupted sutures, using USP 2 chromic catgut or USP 1 polydioxanone) are used to prevent hemorrhage from the vessels in the ileocecal fold. The ligatures are placed near the cecum in order to preserve the vessels supplying the ileum. The ileocecal fold is dissected from distal (cecal apex) to as far

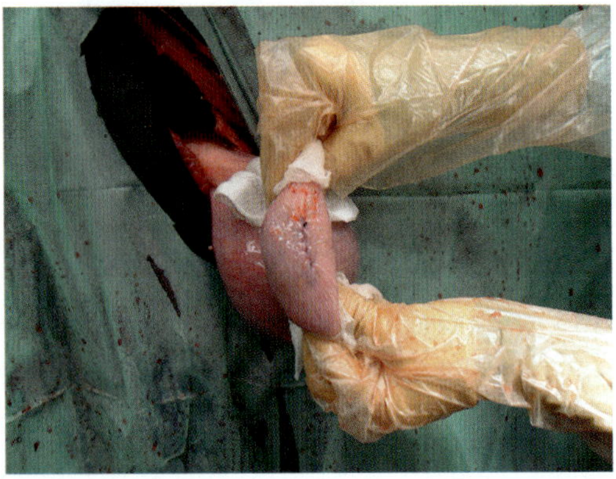

Fig. 4. The cecal apex has been rinsed and closed with a double Cushing suture using 2-0 polyglyconate.

proximal as would be safe to remove the cecal apex without causing abdominal contamination. In the chosen location, two intestinal clamps are placed from the mesenteric and the antimesenteric side of the cecum, through the entire width of the cecal body. The distal part of the cecum is resected 2 to 3 cm distally from the clamps, and the incision is closed in two inverting layers (Cushing or Lembert, with 2-0 polyglyconate or polyglactin 910). The stump is flushed thoroughly with warm saline solution and replaced in the abdominal cavity, which is closed in a routine manner.[7,43] A method with staple closure of the stump was compared with double inverting suture, but the results were not significantly different,[46] and the use of stapling devices in food animals is mostly cost prohibitive. Postoperative care for typhlectomy is the same as that described for typhlotomy.[42] In one study,[43] the long-term prognosis after partial typhlectomy was not better than after simple typhlotomy. Thus, the technically more complicated cecal amputation, resulting in prolonged surgery time and increased degree of contamination, is not recommended as a routine treatment of CDD.[15,43]

Total typhlectomy including removal of the ileocecocolic junction has been performed in experimental[17] and clinical settings,[47] and partial resection of the PLAC has been described;[48] however, these complicated procedures normally require general anesthesia and are unsuitable for treatment of CDD under field conditions.[7]

Prognosis

Except for the risk for recurrence and for peritonitis due to devitalization of the intestinal wall or abdominal contamination at surgery, the prognosis of CDD is considered to be reasonably good, with reports of approximately 90% of referred cases being discharged in good general condition after treatment.[11,42,43] Up to 10% of treated animals will show recurrence of the disease within the first week after typhlotomy and another 12.5% within the first year after surgery.[15,43]

SURGERY OF THE BOVINE COLON

Difficult mobilization and exteriorization of the bovine colon preclude extensive surgical interventions under field conditions. Intussusceptions involving the large intestine (colon or cecum) have been reported predominantly in young animals.[49–52] This condition is presumed to be more common in calves than in adult animals because of the thin colonic mesentery of young animals that allows for more extensive movement of adjacent intestinal segments, in contrast to more extensive mesenteric fat deposits, which stabilize the large intestine in adults.[49,51,53]

Trichobezoars, phytobezoars, and enteroliths, although they mostly lead to disease in the rumen, abomasum, or small intestine, can also cause obstruction of the bovine spiral colon. Clinical signs are similar to those of CDD and a definitive diagnosis is made on abdominal exploration through right flank celiotomy. In such cases, the affected intestinal segment is exteriorized and opened, and the bezoars removed. The enterotomy site is closed with two inverting continuous sutures (Lembert or Cushing [eg, with 3-0 or 2-0 polyglyconate]) apposed transversally if necessary to maximize lumen and prevent stricture formation.[54] Colonic obstruction may further be caused by extraluminal compression (eg, due to adhesions from prior surgery or to mesenteric fat necrosis) (**Fig. 5**). Bypass of the obstruction by side-to-side anastomosis of the bowel proximal to the obstruction and the outer loop of the spiral colon has been described.[7] Two cases of obstruction of the descending colon caused by cecal incarceration in a mesocolic defect in cows have also been described.[55,56]

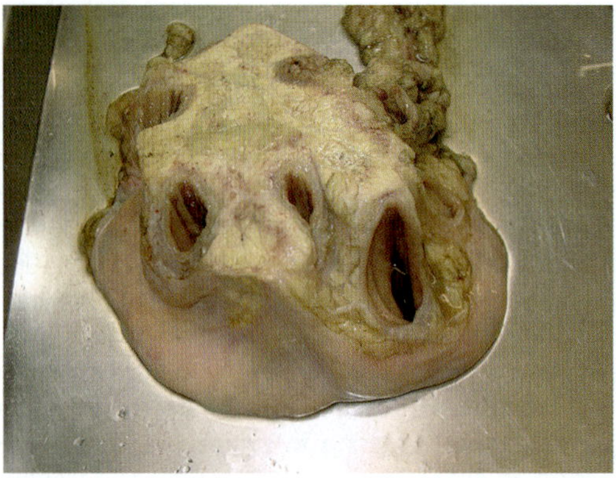

Fig. 5. Loops of the spiral colon embedded in a mass of necrotic fat, which had caused large intestinal obstruction in an Angus cow.

ATRESIA OF THE LARGE INTESTINE

Clinical Presentation and Diagnosis

Atresia of the large intestine (ie, complete occlusion of the intestinal lumen due to abnormal development of the intestinal wall) is a common congenital defect in calves, and numerous descriptions can be found in the literature. This malformation is most commonly seen in the colon of calves, but atresia recti and ani are also of clinical relevance. Atresia of the small intestine, especially of the jejunum, has also been described but is distinctly less common than large intestinal atresia.[57–64] Colonic atresia, mostly encountered in the spiral part of the colon,[53,58–60] has been classified into four types in humans. In type I, the ingesta passage is only hindered by a fold of mucosa occluding the lumen of an otherwise normally developed intestinal canal (**Fig. 6**). In contrast, in type II, the proximal part of the colon ends blind and is connected to the distal segment by a fibrous band devoid of lumen. Type III is similar to type II, but the proximal and the distal intestinal segments are completely separated and a mesenteric defect is present at the level of the atretic segment. Type IV, with

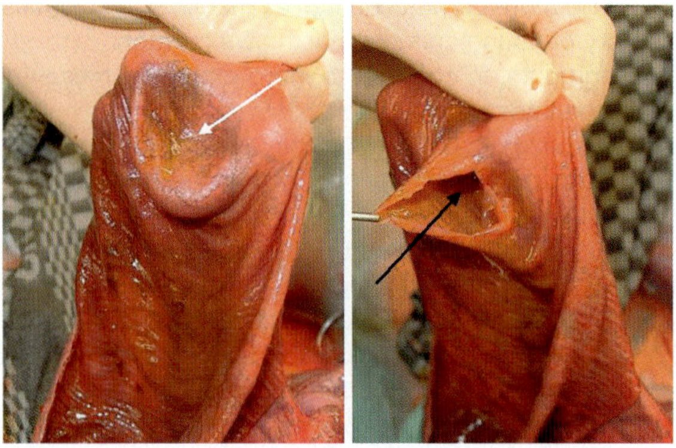

Fig. 6. Type I atresia in the intestine of a 3-day-old Holstein calf. The lumen is completely obstructed by a membrane, the proximal part of the intestine is greatly dilated (*left, white arrow*). After the membrane has been cut open, the lumen of the distal part of the intestine is visible beyond the membrane (*right, black arrow*).

several sites of atresia, is described by some investigators as occurring only in humans.[53,60,63,65–67]

Calves that have large intestinal atresia are typically presented to a veterinarian at the age of 2 or 3 days (although presentation of calves as old as 11 days has been reported), with a history of having been alert and nursing well immediately after birth, but showing decreasing appetite, increasing abdominal discomfort and distention, and progressive weakness after 24 to 36 hours of life. The calves' owners often report that defecation has not been observed since birth. At physical examination, these animals show signs of colic (restlessness, saw-bock stance, kicking toward the abdomen), a distended abdomen, an elevated heart rate, positive percussion and succussion auscultation of the right flank, and neither spontaneous nor provoked defecation. Whereas the absence of an anal opening is immediately visible at physical examination of calves that have atresia ani (**Fig. 7**), the rectum is empty at palpation or contains only mucus in colonic atresia, or can be obstructed at a variable distance from the anus if rectal atresia is present.[57,59–64,68] The dilated rectum protrudes in the perineal region at abdominal palpation in the case of anal atresia alone.[57,61,64] Ultrasonographic examination of the right flank, showing dilated loops of small and large intestine without contractions or movement of ingesta, confirms the diagnosis of ileus (**Fig. 8**). In protracted cases, dilated loops of intestine can be detected by adspection and manual palpation of the right flank.[62] Attempts to confirm a diagnosis of colonic atresia by introducing a catheter from the rectum into the colon to localize the obstruction site should be discouraged because of the risk for perforating the fragile rectal wall of neonates.[2,62,63] Abdominal radiography confirms gas distention of the intestine but even contrast radiography usually does not allow one to identify the atretic area.[61,62,68] Definitive confirmation of the diagnosis occurs at exploratory celiotomy (**Fig. 9**).[59,61,64,68] Because atresia ani is often observed in combination with a malformation or malformations of other parts of the large intestine, a careful, complete physical examination must be performed. Furthermore, if multiple defects are suspected (eg, if abdominal palpation does not induce perineal bulging, suggesting atresia recti in addition to atresia ani), detailed examination of the intestine through celiotomy is indicated before surgery for anal reconstruction.[57,61,64] In some cases of anal atresia in female animals, a rectovaginal fistula develops that allows for defecation through the vagina. In these cases, the animals may be presented much later to the veterinarian because the malformation does not become evident immediately after birth.[57,61]

Hematologic and blood chemistry panels may be normal or may indicate dehydration (elevated packed cell volume or, in advanced cases, signs of prerenal uremia),

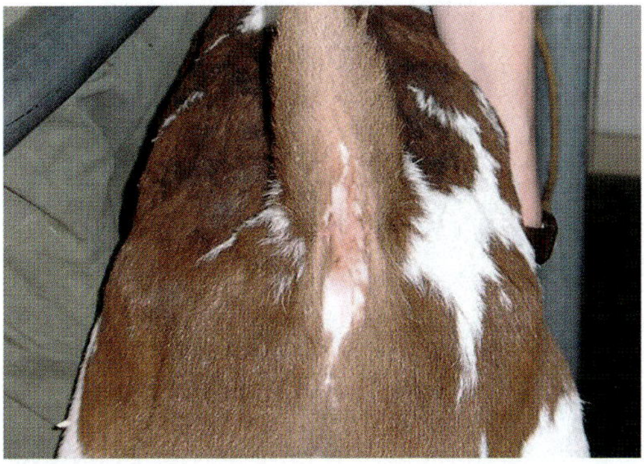

Fig. 7. Atresia ani in a Red Holstein calf.

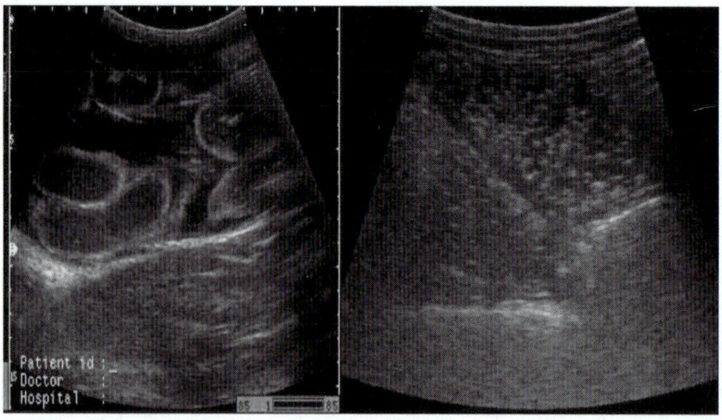

Fig. 8. Typical ultrasonographic findings in the right flank of a calf that has atresia coli, showing dilated small intestines and increased abdominal fluid ventrally (*left*), and dilated loops of large intestine with a cuboidal shape dorsally (*right*). (*Courtesy of* A. Steiner, Dr med vet, FVH, MS, Dr habil, Berne, Switzerland.)

intestinal obstruction (as manifested by hypochloremic, hypokalemic metabolic alkalosis), or in the case of cardiovascular shock or intestinal devitalization, signs of toxemia and metabolic acidosis. Leukocytosis with neutrophilia and left-shift is commonly observed in calves that have atresia coli, but no correlation is evident between white cell count and outcome.[62] Hypogammaglobulinemia is a common finding in calves that have atresia coli, because colostrum ingestion does not necessarily result in absorption of immunoglobulins in calves that have intestinal obstruction.[2,53,59–62]

Differential diagnoses for large intestinal atresia include atresia of the small intestine and, at least in theory, other causes of ileus. However, when the typical combination of anamnesis and clinical presentation described above is present, intestinal malformation must be considered the most likely diagnosis until proved otherwise. A case for

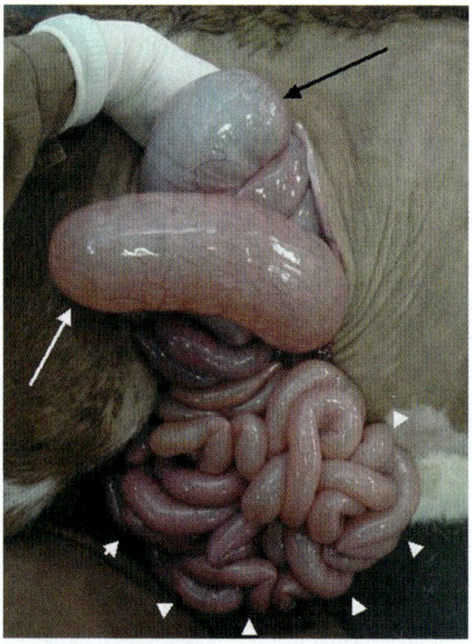

Fig. 9. Atresia coli in a 4-day-old Red Holstein calf with the dilated cecum (*white arrow*), the blind end of the dilated proximal part of the spiral colon (*black arrow*), and dilated small intestine loops (*white arrowheads*). (*Courtesy of* A. Steiner, Dr med vet, FVH, MS, Dr habil, Berne, Switzerland.)

which another cause of ileus would have been found on explorative surgery has not been documented at the Clinic for Ruminants of the Vetsuisse Faculty of Berne during the last 20 years.

Etiopathogenesis

In humans, hereditary factors leading to failure in fetal intestinal development and disruption of the blood supply to the affected portion of the intestine have been discussed as potential causes of intestinal atresia. Intestinal atresia has been reproduced experimentally in dogs and rabbits through in utero ligation of mesenteric vessels.[65] In calves, however, the pathogenesis of intestinal atresia is unknown.[61,64,69,70] The proximal blind end of the colon was examined histologically after surgical resection in nine calves, but no consistent alteration of the intestinal wall was observed.[60] Genetic and traumatic causes have been discussed for intestinal atresia in calves.[58,63,69,71] A genetic component appears to play a role in certain breeds,[71–73] but a report of atresia coli in only one of two identical Simmental twins does not support the hypothesis of a genetic cause, at least in that case.[74] Planned mating experiments with putative carrier dams and sires were suggestive of an autosomal recessive mode of inheritance in the Holstein breed.[72] On the other hand, early pregnancy diagnosis after 35 to 42 days of gestation through palpation of the amniotic vesicle has been suspected of causing disruption of the embryonic vasculature, leading to atresia of intestinal segments.[61,62,69,71,72] Several investigators have observed higher frequency rates of intestinal atresia in calves if amniotic palpation for pregnancy diagnosis had been performed on their dams;[58,71,75] however, in one case, palpation had taken place not before 40 days but between 55 and 90 days of gestation.[62]

Treatment

Anal reconstruction for atresia ani can be performed under epidural anesthesia, with or without sedation. After surgical preparation of the area, a 2.5- to 3-cm–diameter circular piece of skin is removed 4 to 6 cm ventral to the tail, where bulging of the perineum is observed at abdominal palpation. Subcutaneous tissues are prepared bluntly until the meconium-filled rectum can be identified and mobilized. The rectal submucosa is first sutured to subcutaneous perineal tissue in a simple interrupted pattern (2-0 polyglactin 910 or polydioxanone), starting with 4 sutures at 180° and 90° to ensure accurate circumferential alignment. Further adaptation sutures are set subcutaneously as needed and finally, a circular piece of the rectal blind end is excised approximately 1 cm central from the sutures. Skin and full-thickness rectum wall are then apposed in a simple interrupted pattern (0 or 2-0 polypropylene).[53,61,64] Skin incision using a cruciate pattern (instead of resection of a circular piece of skin) leads to anal stricture and is not recommended.[61]

A tentative diagnosis of atresia coli must be confirmed through explorative celiotomy. If the owner refuses surgery, affected calves must be euthanized immediately, before the condition leads to death through autointoxication, circulatory failure, or fecal peritonitis following intestinal rupture. Conservative treatment should not be attempted.

For surgery, the calves are positioned in left lateral recumbency and the right flank is prepared surgically. Depending on the planned intervention (exploratory laparotomy only for diagnosis confirmation before euthanasia, colostomy, or anastomosis of the intestinal blind end to the descending colon), the right paralumbar fossa is anesthetized (eg, with an inverted L-block) or general anesthesia is performed. In the author's opinion, sedation or general anesthesia are not necessary and not recommended for exploratory celiotomy in neonates that have pre-existing cardiovascular compromise, but inhalation anesthesia has been described as the method of choice if anastomosis is to be attempted.[61–63] Preoperative care includes the administration of antibiotics (eg, Na-penicillin, 30,000 IU/kg or a broad-spectrum antibiotic) and intravenous fluids to correct acid-base and electrolyte abnormalities, and non-steroidal anti-inflammatory drugs (eg, flunixin meglumine, 2 mg/g intravenously) as needed. The abdominal cavity is opened routinely[2] but with special caution because the abdominal wall of neonatal calves is thin and, in the case of intestinal atresia, additionally distended by the dilated intestine lying immediately underneath the peritoneum in the right flank. Puncture and gas aspiration for decompression of the intestine may be necessary before exploration of the abdomen can be performed.[62] Colonic atresia is easily diagnosed when a second dilated blind end (of the atretic colon) is found in addition to the dilated cecum (see **Fig. 9**). It is obviously of uppermost relevance to differentiate between the different types of colonic atresia (eg, between type II and type IV) before attempting surgical correction, because the type of malformation will impact not only on surgical options for a given case but also on prognosis for the animal. Furthermore, a thorough exploration of the abdominal cavity is indicated because malformations in other parts of the intestine or in other organs (eg, in the urogenital tract) have been associated with atresia coli.[62]

Four options can be considered after a diagnosis of colonic atresia is confirmed on exploratory surgery: end-to-side or side-to side anastomosis of the proximal blind end of the colon and the colon descendens, end-to-end anastomosis of the intestine proximal and distal to the atretic segment, colostomy, and euthanasia. End-to-end anastomosis is only possible in rare cases because the distal part of the colon is, in most cases, atrophied and cannot be mobilized for end-to-end apposition and suture. Prior to anastomosis, an enterotomy must be performed at the apex of the cecum or the blind end of the proximal colon segment to drain intestinal contents, to reduce tension before attempted anastomosis, and to minimize the possibility of postoperative obstruction through impacted ingesta. The cecal apex or blind end of the colon is exteriorized, and meconium is milked out of the proximal intestine through a stab incision. The enterotomy site is flushed with warm saline solution and closed using a double inverting suture pattern (Cushing or Lembert) and absorbable suture material (eg, 3-0 polyglyconate or polydioxanone). If apposition of the proximal and the distal part of the colon is possible, intestinal clamps are placed across the proximal and distal intestinal segments, the blind ends are removed, and end-to-end anastomosis is performed with absorbable suture material (eg, 3-0 polyglyconate) by first apposing the mesenteric and antimesenteric edges of the intestine with a single perforating simple suture each, and then closing the intestinal lumen either with a double layer of interrupted continuous inverting sutures (Cushing or Lembert) or with a single row of simple perforating interrupted sutures. Surgery to create a bypass of the affected intestinal segment through side-to-side or end-to-side anastomosis between the blind end of the proximal intestinal segment and the descending colon has been described in numerous reports.[2,53,60–62] It is a delicate operation that needs to be performed under general anesthesia.[2] For this procedure, a soft flexible tube can be passed with caution 10 to 20 cm into the rectum by an assistant to allow intra-abdominal identification of the descending colon. A low-volume enema may be administered carefully to remove mucus and cellular debris.[61–63] An intestinal clamp is placed on the proximal colon segment and its blind end is resected. For end-to-side anastomosis, an adequate site is chosen on the descending colon and two simple interrupted Lembert traction sutures are placed approximately 5 cm apart through the antimesenteric seromuscular layer of the descending colon and at 180° intervals on the open proximal colonic segment. The lumen of the descending colon is opened between the stay sutures and end-to-side anastomosis is performed with a single layer of sutures placed in a simple interrupted pattern (with absorbable suture material such as 3-0 polydioxanone, polyglyconate, or polyglactin 910). If necessary, a second layer of inverting sutures is added.[63] If side-to-side anastomosis is to be performed, the transected end of the spiral colon is sutured with a double inverting suture pattern and side-to-side anastomosis is performed in a manner similar to that described earlier for end-to-side anastomosis. The use of stapling devices for colocolic anastomosis has also been described.[53,60,61,63] Some investigators have recommended removing 6 to 10 cm of the dilated proximal blind end of the intestine to prevent anastomotic aperistalsis subsequently to chronic distention,[60,61,63,65] but this procedure did not appear to improve the short-term results of surgery.[63] After completion of the anastomosis, the intestine is flushed carefully with warm saline solution and repositioned in the abdomen. The body wall is closed in a routine manner.

If colostomy is chosen by the surgeon or the owner, or if this salvage procedure is the only possible option because the proximal and distal parts of the intestine cannot be apposed for anastomosis, the blind end of the proximal segment of the intestine is sutured to the skin in 3 layers in the right flank distally to the surgical incision. Localization of the stoma dorsally in the flank results in severe fecal contamination of the abdominal wall, whereas a more ventral stoma bears an increased risk for intestinal prolapse. A circular piece of skin with a diameter of 3 to 4 cm is removed in the chosen location and the muscles of the abdominal wall are prepared by blunt dissection down to the peritoneum. After opening the abdominal cavity, the peritoneum and transverse abdominal muscle are sutured to the skin on both sides of the wound with a size 0 absorbable material to protect the abdominal wall. Then, the blind end of the intestine is pulled through the incision, and the wall of the intestine is sutured to the skin with eight simple interrupted sutures (eg, 0 polyglyconate). The lumen is opened and the intestinal wall is sewn to the skin in a simple continuous pattern.[2,57] As an alternative to the blind end of the proximal segment of the colon, the cecal apex can be sutured to the skin. In such cases, amputation of the colon is recommended to limit impaction of its blind end.[2,68]

In all cases, postoperative care after correction of large intestinal atresia includes antibiotics for at least 5 days (eg, procaine penicillin, 30,000 IU/kg intramuscularly or subcutaneously once daily, or a broad-spectrum antibiotic) and anti-inflammatory drugs as needed. Correction of dehydration and acid-base and electrolyte imbalances with intravenous infusions of saline or polyionic solutions containing glucose has been described by several investigators as an essential part of the clinical management of calves that have intestinal atresia. Plasma administration is indicated in the case of failure of passive transfer of immunity.[2,60–64]

Feces are usually passed within 24 hours of surgery, which are first of loose consistency and become more consistent within 4 to 5 days. Oral feeding can be restored within the first 24 hours after surgery if the calf passed feces, with small amounts of milk or milk replacers fed four to six times daily.[60,63]

Prognosis

The prognosis for atresia ani after surgical correction is principally good if the animals are presented for treatment before they become strongly debilitated and if no anal stricture develops. Although this procedure can be used for salvage, it remains questionable as to whether such animals should be further used for breeding because a genetic component of the development of intestinal atresia is not excluded.[57,61] In addition to combined atresia of multiple intestinal segments, congenital malformations affecting the umbilicus, the urogenital system, the musculoskeletal system, or the eyes have been reported in 18% to 38% of calves that had intestinal atresia.[60,61,63,76]

Short-term survival rates as high as 71% but also as low as 27% have been reported for colonic atresia, and long-term success rates (ie, the percentage of calves born with colonic atresia corrected surgically and subsequently reaching reproductive age) are distinctly lower, ranging from 14.3% to 16.7%.[61–63] In two case series, between 42% and 48% of calves that had atresia coli could be released from the clinic after treatment. The most common postoperative complications were peritonitis secondary to anastomosis failure and megacolon or impaction of the anastomosis despite patent lumen.[60,62] Loose manure and poor growth have been reported in calves after surgery for correction of colon atresia.[60,63] Higher success rates (43%–72%) have been reported for the bypass procedure than for end-to-end anastomosis of the proximal and distal parts of the intestine (17%–40%).[60,63] The prognosis for survival is better for calves that are alert and able to stand at presentation than in severely debilitated calves.[62,64,68]

In one study,[64] creation of a stoma in the flank was unsuccessful in seven out of seven cases; thus, this method should not be recommended. If it should be performed despite these recommendations, calves that have fistulas must be slaughtered when they reach a weight of 130 to 150 kg, to avoid later complications.[2,68]

Because of issues related to animal welfare, because of the high frequency of multiple malformations in calves that have atresia coli,[57,60,63,64] and because the role of genetic inheritability in bovine intestinal atresia is unclear and therefore the impact of continued breeding of such animals on persistence of the malformation in the population is unknown,[73] the author does not recommend surgical correction of colonic atresia. When this diagnosis is confirmed on exploratory surgery at the author's clinic, the calf is usually euthanized immediately after informed consent has been obtained from the owner.

SUMMARY

Surgery for correction of CDD can be performed easily under field conditions, even if cecal amputation needs to be performed. However, complicated cases requiring bypass procedures in the large intestine require general anesthesia and are best performed in hospital conditions.

In calves that have atresia coli, the author recommends celiotomy for confirmation of the diagnosis but not for surgical correction of the condition because of reasons of animal welfare and breeding hygiene. If, however, corrective surgery should be attempted, colostomy can be performed in the field, but the more complicated anastomosis procedures are best done in hospital settings. Anal reconstruction can be performed easily under epidural anesthesia and may allow fattening and salvage of calves born with anal atresia.

REFERENCES

1. Van Metre DC, Callan RJ, Holt TN, et al. Abdominal emergencies in cattle. Vet Clin North Am Food Anim Pract 2005;21:655–96.
2. Mulon PY, Desrochers A. Surgical abdomen of the calf. Vet Clin North Am Food Anim Pract 2005;21:101–32.
3. Meylan M, Eicher R, Steiner A. [Physical examination of ruminants showing signs of abdominal pain]. Schweiz Arch Tierheilkd 1999;141:391–5 [in German].
4. Nickel R, Schummer A, Seiferle E. Eingeweide. In: Schummer A, Nickel R, editors. Lehrbuch der Anatomie der Haustiere. 5th edition. Berlin und Hamburg (Germnay): Paul Parey; 1982. p. 169–77.

5. Maala CP, Sack WO. The arterial supply to the ileum, cecum and proximal loop of the ascending colon in the ox. Anat Histol Embryol 1981;10:130–46.
6. Maala CP, Sack WO. The venous supply of the cecum, ileum, and the proximal loop of the ascending colon in the ox. Anat Histol Embryol 1983;12:154–66.
7. Fubini SL. Surgery of the bovine large intestine. Vet Clin North Am Food Anim Pract 1990;6:461–71.
8. Eicher R, Audige L, Braun U, et al. [Epidemiology and risk factors of cecal dilatation/dislocation and abomasal displacement in dairy cows]. Schweiz Arch Tierheilkd 1999;141:423–9 [in German].
9. Radostits OM. Torsion of the cecum in cattle. Can Vet J 1960;1:405–7.
10. Espersen G. Cecal dilatation and dislocation. Mod Vet Pract 1961;25–7.
11. Dirksen G. [Caecal dilatation and torsion in cattle]. Deutsche Tierärztliche Wochenschrift 1962;15:409–16 [in German].
12. Pearson H. Dilatation and torsion of the bovine caecum and colon. Vet Rec 1963; 75:961–4.
13. Dietz O, Prietz G. [Experience as to the occurrence, diagnosis, and therapy of right abomasal dislocation and cecal dilation and torsion in cattle]. Monatshefte für Veterinärmedizin 1968;23:773–9 [in German].
14. Grunder HD. [Possibilities of conservative treatment of cecum dilatation and torsion in cattle]. Deutsche Tierärztliche Wochenschrift 1971;78:317–9 [in German].
15. Fubini SL, Erb HN, Rebhun WC, et al. Cecal dilatation and volvulus in dairy cows: 84 cases (1977–1983). J Am Vet Med Assoc 1986;189:96–9.
16. Braun U, Eicher R, Hausammann K. Clinical findings in cattle with dilatation and torsion of the caecum. Vet Rec 1989;125:265–7.
17. Maala CP, Smith DF, Hintz HF, et al. Removal of the cecum, including the ileocecocolic junction, and its effects on digestibility in cattle. Am J Vet Res 1983;44: 2237–43.
18. Braun U, Amrein E, Koller U, et al. Ultrasonographic findings in cows with dilatation, torsion and retroflexion of the caecum. Vet Rec 2002;150:75–9.
19. Braun U. Ultrasound as a decision-making tool in abdominal surgery in cows. Vet Clin North Am Food Anim Pract 2005;21:33–53.
20. Braun U, Hermann M, Pabst B. Haematological and biochemical findings in cattle with dilatation and torsion of the caecum. Vet Rec 1989;125:396–8.
21. Muller W. [Cattle cecal dilatation and torsion]. Schweiz Arch Tierheilkd 1970;112: 117–24 [in German].
22. Svendsen P, Kristensen B. Cecal dilatation in cattle. Nord Vet Med 1970;22: 578–83.
23. Stocker S, Steiner A, Geiser S, et al. Myoelectric activity of the cecum and proximal loop of the ascending colon in cows after spontaneous cecal dilatation/dislocation. Am J Vet Res 1997;58:961–8.
24. Steiner A, Roussel AJ, Brumbaugh GW, et al. Myoelectric activity of the cecum and proximal loop of the ascending colon in cows. Am J Vet Res 1994;55: 1037–43.
25. Kobel B, Engel L, Ontsouka EC, et al. Quantitative mRNA analysis of adrenergic receptor subtypes in the intestines of healthy dairy cows and dairy cows with cecal dilatation-dislocation. Am J Vet Res 2006;67:1367–76.
26. Engel L, Kobel B, Ontsouka EC, et al. Distribution of mRNA coding for 5-hydroxytryptamine receptor subtypes in the intestines of healthy dairy cows and dairy cows with cecal dilatation-dislocation. Am J Vet Res 2006;67: 95–101.

27. Ontsouka EC, Steiner A, Bruckmaier RM, et al. Quantitative mRNA analysis of muscarinic acetylcholine receptors in the intestine of dairy cows with spontaneous caecal dilatation-dislocation. Vet J 2008; in press.
28. Ward JK, Richardson D, Tsien WS. Volatile fatty acid concentration and proportions in the gastrointestinal tract of full-fed beef heifers. J Anim Sci 1961;20: 830–2.
29. Siciliano-Jones J, Murphy MR. Production of volatile fatty acids in the rumen and cecum-colon of steers as affected by forage:concentrate and forage physical form. J Dairy Sci 1989;72:485–92.
30. Matthé A, Lebzien P, Flachowski G. Zur Dedeutung von Bypass-Stärke für die Glucoseversorgung von hochleistenden Milchkühen. Übersichten zur Tierernährung 2000;28:1–64.
31. Breves G, Diener M, Ehrlein HJ, et al. Physiologie des Magen-Darm-Kanals. In: von Engelhardt W, Breves B, editors. Physiologie der Haustiere. Stuttgart (Germany): Enke im Hyppokrates Verlag GmbH; 2000. p. 303–407.
32. Svendsen P. Inhibition of cecal motility in sheep by volatile fatty acids. Nord Vet Med 1972;24:393–6.
33. Svendsen P. Abomasal displacement in cattle. Nord Vet Med 1970;22:571–7.
34. Bolton JR, Merritt AM, Carlson GM, et al. Normal abomasal electromyography and emptying in sheep and the effects of intraabomasal volatile fatty acid infusion. Am J Vet Res 1976;37:1387–92.
35. Gregory PC. Inhibition of reticulo-ruminal motility by volatile fatty acids and lactic acid in sheep. J Physiol 1987;382:355–71.
36. Fioramonti J, Ruckebusch Y. Diet and caecal motility in sheep. Ann Rech Vet 1979;10:593–9.
37. Madison JB, Merritt AM, Rice B, et al. Influence of an abrupt change in diet on antroduodenal myoelectric activity in lactating cattle. Am J Vet Res 1993;54: 793–7.
38. Lester GD, Bolton JR. Effect of dietary composition on abomasal and duodenal myoelectrical activity. Res Vet Sci 1994;57:270–6.
39. Abegg R, Eicher R, Lis J, et al. Concentration of volatile fatty acids in digesta samples obtained from healthy cows and cows with cecal dilatation or dislocation. Am J Vet Res 1999;60:1540–5.
40. Allemann M, Eicher R, Mevissen M, et al. Effect of sodium butyric acid, sodium valerianic acid, and osmolarity on contractility of specimens of intestinal wall obtained from the cecum and spiral colon of healthy cows. Am J Vet Res 2000; 61:678–83.
41. Meylan M, Eicher R, Blum JW, et al. Effects of an abrupt increase of starch-rich concentrates in the diet of dairy cows on concentrations of volatile fatty acids in the rumen and large intestine and on myoelectric activity of the spiral colon. Am J Vet Res 2002;63:857–67.
42. Braun U, Steiner A, Bearth G. Therapy and clinical progress of cattle with dilatation and torsion of the caecum. Vet Rec 1989;125:430–3.
43. Steiner A, Braun U, Lischer C, et al. Surgical treatment of cecal dilatation/torsion in the cow 80 cases (1988–1990). [Die chirurgische Behandlung der Blinddarm-dilatation/-torsion bei der Kuh–80 Fälle (1988-1990)]. Wien Tierärztl Monatsschr 1992;79:41–6 [in German].
44. Steiner A, Meylan M, Eicher R. [New aspects on the etiopathogenesis and treatment of cecal dilatation/-dislocation in cows-a review]. Schweiz Arch Tierheilkd 1999;141:419–22 [in German].

45. Tulleners EP. Prevention and treatment of complications of bovine gastrointestinal surgery. Vet Clin North Am Food Anim Pract 1990;6:495–514.
46. Steiner A, Braun U, Waldvogel A. Comparison of staple and suture techniques for partial typhlectomy in the cow: a prospective clinical study of 40 cases. Zentralbl Veterinarmed A 1992;39:26–37.
47. Green MJ, Husband JA. Sigmoid caecal volvulus in a dairy cow treated by total typhlectomy. Vet Rec 1996;139:233–5.
48. Pankowski RL, Fubini SL, Stehman S. Cecal volvulus in a dairy cow: partial resection of the proximal portion of the ascending colon. J Am Vet Med Assoc 1987; 191:435–6.
49. Horne MM. Colonic intussusception in a Holstein calf. Can Vet J 1991;32:493–5.
50. Hamilton GF, Tulleners EP. Intussusception involving the spiral colon in a calf. Can Vet J 1980;21:32.
51. Constable PD, St Jean G, Hull BL, et al. Intussusception in cattle: 336 cases (1964–1993). J Am Vet Med Assoc 1997;210:531–6.
52. Doll K, Klee W, Dirksen G. [Cecal intussusception in calves]. Tierärztl Prax 1998; 26:247–53 [in German].
53. Bristol DG, Fubini SL. Surgery of the neonatal bovine digestive tract. Vet Clin North Am Food Anim Pract 1990;6:473–93.
54. Anderson DE, Ewoldt JM. Intestinal surgery of adult cattle. Vet Clin North Am Food Anim Pract 2005;21:133–54.
55. Ross MW, Ducharme NG, Power HT. Torsion of the descending colon in a cow. Can Vet J 1983;24:150–1.
56. Diefenderfer DL, Tulleners EP. Obstruction of the descending colon due to torsion of the cecum through a mesocolic defect in a cow. J Am Vet Med Assoc 1986; 188:1440–1.
57. Steenhaut M, De Moor A, Verschooten F, et al. Intestinal malformations in calves and their surgical correction. Vet Rec 1976;98:131–3.
58. Ness H, Leopold G, Müller W. Genesis of congenital ileus in calf (atresia coli et jejuni). [Zur Genese des angeborenen Darmverschlusses (Atresia coli et jejuni) des Kalbes]. Monatshefte für Veterinärmedizin 1982;37:89–92 [in German].
59. Johnson R, Ames NK, Coy C. Congenital intestinal atresia of calves. J Am Vet Med Assoc 1983;182:1387–9.
60. Ducharme NG, Arighi M, Horney FD, et al. Colonic atresia in cattle: a prospective study of 43 cases. Can Vet J 1988;29:818–24.
61. Dreyfuss DJ, Tulleners EP. Intestinal atresia in calves: 22 cases (1978–1988). J Am Vet Med Assoc 1989;195:508–13.
62. Constable PD, Rings DM, Hull BL, et al. Atresia coli in calves: 26 cases (1977–1987). J Am Vet Med Assoc 1989;195:118–23.
63. Smith DF, Ducharme NG, Fubini SL, et al. Clinical management and surgical repair of atresia coli in calves: 66 cases (1977–1988). J Am Vet Med Assoc 1991;199:1185–90.
64. Martens A, Gasthuys F, Steenhaut M, et al. Surgical aspects of intestinal atresia in 58 calves. Vet Rec 1995;136:141–4.
65. Louw JH. Congenital intestinal atresia and stenosis in the newborn. Observations on its pathogenesis and treatment. Ann R Coll Surg Engl 1959;25:209–34.
66. van der Gaag I, Tibboel D. Intestinal atresia and stenosis in animals: a report of 34 cases. Vet Pathol 1980;17:565–74.
67. Johnson R. Intestinal atresia and stenosis: a review comparing its morphology. Vet Res Commun 1986;10:105–11.

68. Berchtold M, Mittelholzer A, Camponovo L. [Colonic atresia in the calf]. Deutsche Tierärztliche Wochenschrift 1985;92:395–8 [in German].
69. Johnson R. Intestinal atresia and stenosis: a review comparing its etiopathogenesis. Vet Res Commun 1986;10:95–104.
70. Saperstein G. Congenital abnormalities of internal organs and body cavities. Vet Clin North Am Food Anim Pract 1993;9:115–25.
71. Syed M, Shanks RD. Incidence of atresia coli and relationships among the affected calves born in one herd of Holstein cattle. J Dairy Sci 1992;75:1357–64.
72. Syed M, Shanks RD. Atresia coli inherited in Holstein cattle. J Dairy Sci 1992;75:1105–11.
73. Syed M, Shanks RD. What causes atresia coli in Holstein calves? Cornell Vet 1993;83:261–3.
74. Hoffsis GF, Bruner RR Jr. Atresia coli in a twin calf. J Am Vet Med Assoc 1977;171:433–4.
75. Brenner J, Orgad U. Epidemiological investigations of an outbreak of intestinal atresia in two Israeli dairy herds. J Vet Med Sci 2003;65:141–3.
76. Sharratt RK. The surgical correction of a case of anorectal agenesis in a calf. Vet Rec 1966;79:108–10.

Unilateral Nephrectomy of Cattle

Matt D. Miesner, DVM, MS*, David E. Anderson, DVM, MS

KEYWORDS

• Bovine • Cattle • Nephrectomy • Kidney • Renal
• Pyelonephritis

Renal disease is occasionally diagnosed in cattle. Most often, renal disease is bilateral and medical therapy is the treatment of choice. Nephrectomy may be performed in selected cases where a single kidney is primarily involved and medical therapy is unsuccessful. Unilateral nephrectomy can be performed successfully in affected cattle; this surgery can be performed under field settings, and these cattle can remain productive members of the herd. Examples of these cases include polycystic kidney, unilateral renal abscess, unilateral renal neoplasia, unilateral ureteral obstruction, and other such injuries. The most common renal injury in our experience is associated with urinary tract infection.

Urinary tract infection (UTI) in food animals, like other species, results most commonly from ascending infection of pathogenic bacteria normally inhabiting the genitourinary epithelium and gastrointestinal tract, or residing in the environment. Infection may ascend proximal from the bladder to include unilateral or bilateral disease of the ureters and kidneys. Left sided pyelonephritis is most commonly diagnosed clinically although bilateral disease may be present. Hematogenous spread is reported much less frequently, but possible. Ascending infection may originate from the lower urinary tract, much more likely in females, and is often reported with a history of decreased frequency of urination and with postparturient diseases in cows. Dehydration may result in lower volumes of urine produced and stagnation of urine flow. Downer cows often urinate infrequently, if at all without assistance, and are in closer prolonged proximity to environmental contaminants. Other origins for ascending infection may be from an infected urachus in neonates, indwelling transabdominal cystostomy tubes or stoma after surgery for urethral obstruction, or introduced through urethral catheterization and obstetric manipulation. Inflammation within the urinary tract, from trauma or urinary calculi, increase the risk of an established UTI, although *Escherichia coli*, *Corynebacterium renale* (cattle), and *Eubacterium suis* (swine) can establish primary infections in normal mucosa.

Department of Clinical Sciences, College of Veterinary Medicine, Kansas State University, 1800 Dennison Avenue, Manhattan, KS 66506, USA
* Corresponding author. Department of Clinical Sciences, Kansas State University, Veterinary Medicine Teaching Hospital,103J Mosier Hall, Manhattan, KS 66506-5701.
E-mail address: mmiesner@vet.k-state.edu (M.D. Miesner).

Vet Clin Food Anim 24 (2008) 497–500
doi:10.1016/j.cvfa.2008.07.002
0749-0720/08/$ – see front matter. Published by Elsevier Inc.

The most commonly isolated organism from pyelonephritis cases in cattle is *E. coli*, followed closely by *C. renale*. *E. coli* would more commonly be considered in the environmental or opportunistic pathogen, whereas *C. renale* is commonly considered the agent of infectious pyelonephritis. Though both can normally reside subclinically in urogenital epithelium, poor on-farm environmental hygiene increases the frequency of clinical disease. *C. renale* are continually disseminated into the environment from infected animals and may survive there for 2 months.[1] Other *Corynebacterium* species, coliforms, and *Arcanobacterium pyogenes* are also capable of causing disease. The ability to isolate *Corynebacterum* species as well as *Eubacterium suis* (formerly *Corynebacterium*) from prepuces of bulls and boars (prepucial diverticulum) makes venereal transmission possible.[2,3]

DIAGNOSIS

In cattle, a history of illthrift, fever, and vague colic signs accompany a diagnosis of pyelonephritis. Careful questioning of the observant owner may also reveal a history of straining to urinate or pus in the urine. Often, cattle are diagnosed after a chronic course of disease. *Eubacterium suis* infections in swine may present as either a chronic disease or a short course of acute disease and death in less than a few days.

Physical examination of cattle with suspected pyelonephritis should include urinalysis for evidence of hematuria, leukouria, bacteriuria, and proteinuria. Isosthenuria with an alkaline pH is common. It is important to observe the complete urination period as debris may have settled to the ventral bladder wall and only be voided terminally in the urination process. Rectal examination should determine pain elicited on palpation of the kidneys (usually only the left can be palpated rectally), which may feel enlarged, and decreased lobulations. The ureters can be located at approximately 11 and 1 o'clock anterior to the wings of the ilium, and are retroperitoneal. Normal ureters are the size of a large pencil lead and can be "slipped" between the fingertips. Enlarged ureters can be palpated for enlargement and turgidity. The urinary bladder wall may feel thickened.

Ultrasonography of urinary soft tissues per rectum or kidneys per cutaneous in the paralumbar fossas provides a valuable diagnostic aid for determining the extent or severity of UTI. Ultrasound of the craniodorsal, right paralumbar fossa at the twelfth intercostal space is of particular benefit for determining pathology of the right kidney because palpation per rectum is limited. Findings may reveal dilated renal calices containing hyperechoic debris.[4]

MEDICAL TREATMENT

Antibiotic selection should be based on culture and sensitivity if available; however, penicillin is the most common initial treatment of choice. Overwhelming infection may result in a lack of therapeutic response despite bacterial susceptibility. Long-term antibiotic administration should be recommended, extending at least 4 weeks. Limited studies have suggested relapse rates of nearly 10% and overall mortality or culling rates of one-third of clinical cases.[5] Medical treatment outcome will depend largely on the duration and extent of infection.

Determining bilateral disease is important and extent of renal function is more difficult to determine in ruminants. Measuring urine specific gravity, azotemia response to fluid therapy, and physical examination findings should be combined to determine response to therapy. Nephrectomy may be an option for some individuals, and both kidneys can be carefully evaluated with palpation and ultrasound during the exploratory.

Promoting diuresis is an important adjunctive therapy in flushing the urinary tract. Intravenous fluids may be used initially or in severe cases. Oral fluids through tubing and encouraging water intake should be done. Providing salt and feeding ammonium chloride (maximum of 200 mg/kg per day) will encourage water consumption. Ammonium chloride has the added benefit of urine acidification, which may prevent adhesion of some organisms.

SURGICAL TREATMENT

Persistent unilateral infection or other unilateral renal pathology justifies unilateral nephrectomy in valuable cattle. In the authors' experience, unilateral nephrectomy is most commonly diagnosed in dairy breed cows between 2 and 7 years old, and the left kidney is most commonly affected. The most common clinical signs are decreased appetite, poor milk production, weight loss, diarrhea, pyuria, infertility, lethargy, pollakiuria, hematuria, swelling of the rear limbs, and abdominal distention. Physical examination findings are likely to include fever, tachycardia, renal pain on palpation, and enlarged ureter. Hematology in affected cattle most often reveals mild leukocytosis characterized by a neutrophil:lymphocyte reversal. Cattle with pyelonephritis are characterized by marked hyperfibrinoginemia. Serum biochemistry analysis is indicated because azotemia in the face of normal hydration suggests insufficient renal parenchyma to allow return to productivity because of bilateral renal involvement. If biochemistry reveals normal serum creatinine, blood urea nitrogen, potassium, serum protein, and plasma protein, the cow is judged to be a good surgical candidate for nephrectomy. Urinalysis should be done routinely and surgical candidates have a normal specific gravity and pH of 8, but commonly have proteinuria, hematuria and pyuria. Bacteria are occasionally seen in the urine of pyelonephritis cattle.

Unilateral nephrectomy is most often performed with the cow standing in a restraint chute. Nephrectomy is performed via a standing paralumbar fossae approach in most cattle. The kidney is removed via right paralumbar fossae (right or left kidney) or via left paralumbar fossae. Rarely, nephrectomy is done under general anesthesia. Proximal paravertebral anesthesia is preferred to ensure the largest possible zone of anesthesia. A standard laparotomy incision is made and the dorsal peritoneum incised to provide access to the retroperitoneal space surrounding the kidney. Blunt dissection is used to free the kidney from surrounding tissues and isolate the renal vascular pedicle. Gentle traction is used to expose and isolate the renal artery and vein. Excessive traction may cause the cow to become recumbent, cause acute hypotension, or lead to hemorrhage. After isolating the affected kidney, No. 1 or No. 2 suture (PGA, PG-910, PDS, and so forth) is used to triple ligate the renal artery and vein. If found, the ureter can be ligated using No. 0 suture material. If the ureter is not easily identified, it can be transected with other perirenal tissues and left free within the retroperitoneal space. Death may occur during or immediately after surgery and is most commonly associated with severe hemorrhage. The authors recommend multiple ligatures of size No. 1 or 2 be placed on the renal artery and vein to ensure secure ligation. The laparotomy incision is closed in routine fashion. Perioperatvie care is based on clinical signs and may include antibiotics, anti-inflammatory drugs, intravenous fluids, pain medication, and so forth.

After surgery, cattle are confined for 14 to 21 days before returning to the herd. Urinalysis and serum biochemistry profile during the postoperative period will allow assessment of the function of the remaining kidney. Damage to the remaining kidney suggesting a poor to grave prognosis include hyposthenuria, persistent pyuria or proteinuria, azotemia, or clinical signs of lethargy, inappetence, or poor milk production.

Unilateral nephrectomy is a useful treatment for renal disease in cattle where one kidney is principally involved. Removal of the worst affected kidney has been successful in the authors' experience, with most affected cattle returning to acceptable levels of productivity. However, clients should be aware that performance may be suboptimal. Unilateral nephrectomy is warranted for treatment of affected cattle of perceived high economic value.

REFERENCES

1. Hayashi A, Yangawa R, Kida H. Survival of *Corynebacterium renale* and *Corynebacterium pilosum* and *Corynebacterium cystitidis* in soil. Vet Microbiol 1985;10(4):381–6.
2. Pijoan C, Lastra A, Leman A. Isolation of *Corynebacterium suis* from the prepuce of boars. J Am Vet Med Assoc 1983;183(4):428–9.
3. Tubbs RC. Cystitis, Pyelonephritis, and miscellaneous diseases of swine. In: Howard JL, Smith RA, editors. Current vet therapy: food animal practice, 4th edition. Philadelphia: WB Saunders; 1999. p. 631–2.
4. Hayashi H, Biller DS, Rings DM, et al. Ultrasonographic diagnosis of pyelonephritis in a cow. J Am Vet Med Assoc 1994;205(5):736–8.
5. Markusfeld O, Nahari N, Kessner D, et al. Observations of bovine pyelonephritis in cattle. Br Vet J 1989;145(6):573–9.

Surgical Procedures of the Thorax

David E. Anderson, DVM, MS[a], Guy St. Jean, DMV, MS[b]

KEYWORDS

• Thorax • Trachea • Lung • Diaphragm • Mediastinum

ANATOMY

Extensive anatomic descriptions of the head, neck, and thorax are beyond the scope of this article; however, ruminants have anatomic features that large animal veterinarians should consider when evaluating an animal with lesions affecting the respiratory system. The trachea has a right tracheal bronchus leading to the right cranial lung lobe. This bronchus may be the site of choice for collection of culture and cytology samples in cattle affected by cranioventral bronchopneumonia. In addition, this anatomic feature causes pulmonary diseases to occur more frequently on the right hemi-thorax.

PHYSICAL EXAMINATION

Physical examination of the respiratory system of cattle may be difficult, depending on the nature of the animal.[1–4] Halter-trained cattle are certainly easier to examine than cattle accustomed to the open range. A complete physical examination is critical to thorough work-up of cattle affected with respiratory disease. Determination of the location and severity of the disease is of utmost importance to the surgeon, and will help to narrow the list of differential diagnoses. The character, frequency, and depth of respirations should be noted. In addition, the thorax, trachea, larynx, and paranasal sinuses should be ausculted separately to identify the point of maximal intensity of abnormal sounds. The nares should be felt to determine symmetry of air movement and depth of respiration in proportion to the size of the animal. A specialized mouth speculum has been designed for examination of the caudal oropharynx and larynx of cattle.[5] This speculum simultaneously opens the mouth and depresses the tongue. Thoracic auscultation should be performed for all lung fields on both sides of the thorax. Thoracic acoustic percussion can also contribute significantly to the information database, particularly when thoracic radiographs and ultrasonography are not available.[6] Hematology and serum biochemistry analysis may be indicated to characterize

[a] Department of Clinical Sciences, College of Veterinary Medicine, Kansas State University, 1800 Dennison Avenue, Manhattan, KS 66506, USA
[b] Ross University School of Veterinary Medicine, P.O. Box 334, Basseterre, St. Kitts, West Indies
E-mail address: danderso@vet.ksu.edu (D.E. Anderson).

Vet Clin Food Anim 24 (2008) 501–510
doi:10.1016/j.cvfa.2008.07.004 **vetfood.theclinics.com**
0749-0720/08/$ – see front matter © 2008 Elsevier Inc. All rights reserved.

the nature or severity of a given disease. These tests are chosen after determining economic constraints and when interpretation is believed to be beneficial for guiding therapy or prognosis.

RADIOGRAPHIC EXAMINATION

Radiographic examination is indicated when physical examination has isolated the disease to a specific area but cannot sufficiently determine the nature or severity of the disease. Radiographs are useful for evaluation of the trachea and thorax because the surrounding air density allows detection of soft-tissue pathology. In addition, lesions may be localized to a specific segment of the respiratory system, such as a pulmonary abscess or pericarditis (**Fig. 1**).

ENDOSCOPIC EXAMINATION

When possible, chemical restraint should not be used to facilitate endoscopic examination because significant alteration of the endoscopic anatomy may occur.[7,8] A 1-m long endoscope is sufficient to view the nasal passages, pharynx, larynx, proximal trachea, and esophagus of most adult cattle. The tracheal bronchus can be viewed in most animals less than 700 kg, but a 3-m endoscope may be necessary for examination of the mainstem bronchi and the full length of the esophagus. The upper airway anatomy of cattle differs from that of horses. Therefore, the examiner should be familiar with bovine anatomy. Pigmentation of the pharynx and larynx is not uncommon in cattle, and pigmented areas should not be misinterpreted as pathologic tissues.[7]

ULTRASONOGRAPHIC EXAMINATION

Ultrasonographic examination of the ventral neck and mediastinum has been described for cattle.[9,10] These examinations may be useful to determine the association of abscesses with vital structures, search for foreign bodies, and determine the extent of lesions before surgery. Interpretation of ultrasonographic images is directly proportional to the examiner's knowledge of bovine anatomy and experience level. In one study, thoracic ultrasonography was more sensitive than radiographs for detection of small pleural effusion and pulmonary consolidation.[11]

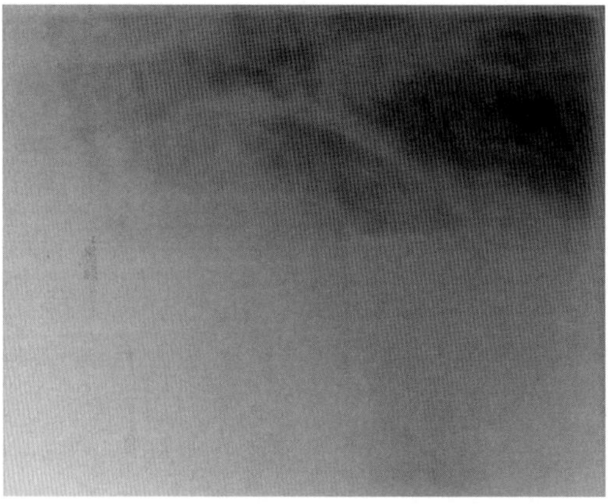

Fig. 1. Thoracic radiograph of a bull with lethargy, anorexia, weight loss, exercise intolerance, and increased jugular pulses. A large confluent gas-fluid interface is apparent and consistent with septic pericarditis (confirmed at necropsy).

Tracheal Collapse

Tracheal collapse is usually seen in young calves exhibiting inspiratory distress. The calves often breathe with the mouth open and head and neck extended.[12,13] Nasal oxygen often improves arterial oxygen pressure and should be used if possible to stabilize the animal. The inspiratory phase is prolonged and a "honking" cough is often present, especially with intrathoracic collapse. In some animals there may be other evidence of trauma, such as fractured ribs.[12,14] There is no response to antibiotics, steroids, or tracheostomy.[13] A history of a progressively worsening inspiratory dyspnea in a calf delivered by forced extraction is good presumptive evidence for tracheal collapse.[15] To confirm the diagnosis a lateral radiograph of the posterior cervical and thoracic trachea should be obtained. Radiographs will also define which segment is affected. A number of treatments have been proposed in cattle as well as other species, including resection and anastomosis, resection of tracheal rings, external prosthesis, and plication of the dorsal membrane.[12–14] Mild cases of tracheal collapse may respond to stall confinement sufficiently until slaughter. The author currently recommends external prosthesis, but a favorable prognosis for this surgery probably exists in no more than 30% of cases.[15] In preparation for surgery, a prosthetic tracheal ring should be constructed. A 35-mL or 60-mL syringe will work well for young calves.[12] Segments of syringe equal to the length of two to four tracheal rings are cut and a small segment of the ring is removed to enable the surgeon to pass the ring around the trachea. Holes are drilled through the prosthetic rings around the circumference to serve as suture points to the prosthesis and the collapsed segments. With the animal under inhalation anesthesia, it is positioned in dorsal recumbency, with the front limbs pulled posterior. A midline skin incision is made from the midcervical area to the manubrium. The cervical muscles are divided by blunt dissection and the trachea exposed. One should note that before the connective tissue surrounding the trachea is dissected, the vagosympathetic trunk should be identified and gently retracted. One or more prosthetic rings may be needed to correct the collapse. A ring is selected, fitted around the trachea, and sutures are prep-laced around the ring. When the three or four sutures have been threaded through the ring, the ring is opposed to the trachea and secured via the suture. When all the knots have been pulled secure around the prosthesis, the trachea should be expanded to the diameter of the prosthesis. The tissues are then opposed over the trachea.

Short- and long-term postoperative complications are common. Dyspnea may be observed after surgery if additional tracheal segments collapse. Because the prosthesis is done on young calves, as the calf grows the tracheal luminal diameter of the affected segment is limited by the size of the prosthesis.[15] Therefore, progressive tracheal stenosis and inspiratory dyspnea may return. Furthermore, when surgical repair was successful long term, affected cattle were smaller when compared with age-matched herd mates. Thus, surgical correction of tracheal collapse is rarely performed because of the guarded to poor long-term outcome for these calves.

Tracheal Stenosis

Tracheal laceration or trauma may cause focal stenosis by fibroplasia and wound contracture. Usually, tracheal stenosis does not cause clinical signs of respiratory problems, and affected cattle are productive members of the herd. Severe tracheal stenosis may cause increased respiratory rate, prolong inspiratory time (increased inoperatory-to-expiratory time ratio), and open-mouth breathing. Affected cattle have decreased appetite, lose weight, and are not productive. Options for surgical correction include excision of granulation tissue, application of a tracheal prosthesis, and tracheal resection and anastomosis. Excision of granulation tissue may be performed transendoscopically or by tracheotomy when the cervical portion of the trachea is involved. Partial tracheal resection and end-to-end anastomosis can be performed for the cervical portion of the trachea. The length of the trachea removed should be strictly minimized. As a rule of thumb, a maximum of three to five tracheal rings may be excised for successful reconstruction of the trachea. Interrupted suture patterns and monofilament suture (# 1 PDS, # 1 Nylon, or other such monofilaments) should be used. Suture material should not enter the lumen of the trachea. A 1.5-year-old heifer suffered severe tracheal stenosis following an attack by a leopard.[16] The heifer developed open-mouth breathing, which had been present for 30 days before surgery. The fourth, fifth and sixth tracheal rings were excised and end-to-end anastomosis performed. Monofilament nylon was used in an interrupted mattress pattern. Radiographs on day 30 after surgery revealed partial tracheal stenosis at the site of the anastomosis, but the heifer was clinically normal. The heifer was able to exercise without becoming dyspneic.

LUNGS

Pulmonary Abscess

Lung abscesses are usually caused by chronic pneumonia, septicemia, or secondary to trauma or parasite infestation. Often, these abscesses are multiple and spread throughout the lung parenchyma. Therefore, surgical treatment is not practical; however, lung abscess secondary to foreign body penetration of the lung (including traumatic reticulopleuritis/pneumonitis) may be amenable to surgery. Surgical treatment of pulmonary abscesses may include partial lung lobectomy or marsupialization of a large abscess. The author has marsupialized a large abscess within the right caudal lung lobe of a 2-year-old Simmental heifer. The abscess was caused by a wire penetrating through the reticulum and into the caudal aspect of the lung. The abscess was identified using ultrasonography and evaluated by thoroscopy. Six centimeters of the overlying seventh rib were resected, and the capsule of the abscess marsupialized to the thoracic wall and skin. These abscesses may contain *A. pyogenes,* F. *necrophorum, Clostridium* spp, and mixed populations of gram-positive and gram-negative bacteria.

Lung Biopsy

Percutaneous lung biopsy has been used in cattle to obtain specimens for cytology, histopathology, bacterial and fungal culture, or for virus isolation.[17] In the author's experience, this technique has limited usefulness compared with transtracheal wash or bronchoalveolar lavage because of the risk of pneumothorax or pleuritis. Pulmonary disease must be regionally diffuse to ensure that a diagnostic specimen is obtained. Furthermore, lung biopsy has the risk of inducing tension pneumothorax, hemothorax, or pyothorax. Lung biopsy can be done through the fifth, sixth, seventh, or eighth intercostal space at a point approximately 10-cm to 15-cm dorsal to the costochondral junction. The author recommends ultrasound guidance or thoroscopy to increase the chances of obtaining a diagnostic specimen. Once the site has been selected, the hair is clipped, aseptically prepared, and local anesthesia induced with 2% lidocaine HCl. Care should be taken not to lacerate the lung with the tip of the needle in case of sudden movement by the animal. Cattle should be observed for respiratory distress (pneumothorax, hemothorax) for 6 to 12 hours after biopsy.

Surgical Approach to the Lung and Mediastinum

Surgery of the lung or mediastinal structures is rarely indicated in cattle. Lung abscesses or congenital anomalies in calves may be removed by lung lobectomy. Collapsing trachea in calves, tracheal foreign body, or intrathoracic esophageal obstruction may require surgical approach to the mediastinum. The cranial rib cage of cattle has limited compliance; therefore, exposure to the cranioventral thorax requires rib resection. Fifth or sixth rib resection and thoracotomy is described under surgery of the thorax. Exposure of the cranial portion of the thoracic trachea is done by resection of the first two ribs from a caudal cervical approach. This surgery is described under surgery of the trachea. Exposure to the caudal lung lobes and mediastinum is done by making a 15 cm long vertical incision into the pleural space through the seventh, eighth, or ninth intercostal space. The incision is begun approximately 10-cm dorsal to the costochondral junction and extended dorsally. The caudal lung lobes are immediately accessible. The mediastinum is approached by cranial displacement of the lungs and careful dissection. Disruption of the vagus and phrenic nerves, the caudal vena cava, descending aorta, or esophagus is undesirable. Positive-pressure ventilation is required when performing thoracotomy with the animal in lateral recumbency. Rib resection can be performed in standing cattle and cattle restrained on an inclined table without mechanical ventilation because of the intact mediastinum; however, the author recommends that immediate access to tracheal intubation and ventilation be available before standing thoracotomy is attempted. The intercostal muscles and pleura are closed together with absorbable suture material (#1 polydioxinone or polymerized caprolactam) and subcutaneous tissues and skin closure is routine.

THORAX AND DIAPHRAGM

Thoracic Wounds, Rib Fracture

Thoracic wounds causing compromise of the thoracic cavity are infrequently found in cattle. Puncture wounds, such as from homed cattle, gunshot, fence posts, or other foreign bodies can cause tension pneumothorax and pyothorax. Tension pneumothorax is created when a wound in the thoracic wall or lung allows movement of air into the pleural space but does not allow exiting of the air. Thus, intrathoracic pressure increases cause collapse of the lung and diminished movement of the diaphragm and thoracic wall. Tension pneumothorax is immediately life threatening. Placement of a chest tube or suction tube into the affected side of the thorax is followed by immediate improvement in respiratory effort. Open thoracic wounds (allowing two-way movement of air) are usually not immediately life threatening because of the complete mediastinum of cattle. Cattle can adequately oxygenate their blood with one healthy lung; however, productivity is markedly compromised. Open wounds may be treated by surgical closure (which may require use of a myocutaneous flap) and re-establishment of normal thoracic pressure by use of a suction tube or one-way valve (Heimlich) attached to a chest tube.

Rib fracture occurs most commonly in calves born with dystocia. Excessive traction during manual extraction of the calf can cause fracture of ribs 1, 2, 3, 4, or 5, or any combination of these. Multiple rib fractures may cause a flail chest-breathing pattern. The rib cage caudal to rib 5 is more compliant, and trauma is less likely to cause fracture during dystocia. Trailer accidents may result in rib fracture, but fracture in the appendicular skeleton is more common. Although calves usually do well in the immediate postparturient period after rib fracture, these calves may succumb to pneumonia or septicemia, or may develop progressive tracheal collapse.

Pleuritis and Pericarditis

In cattle, pericarditis is most commonly caused by penetrating foreign bodies originating in the reticulum. Pleuritis may be caused by pneumonia, pulmonary abscess, extension of a liver abscess through the diaphragm, and penetrating reticular foreign bodies.[18,19] Nonseptic pleural effusion is most commonly caused by heart failure or thoracic neoplasia. Septic pericarditis has a poor-to-grave prognosis for life, and septic pleuritis has a guarded-to-poor prognosis for life. In one retrospective study, cattle with pericarditis (n = 7) or unilateral pleuritis (n = 7) had thoracotomy performed.[18] Of seven cattle with pericarditis, one survived to discharge from the hospital. Of seven cattle with unilateral pleuritis, five survived to discharge from the hospital. One year after discharge, five cows were productive and one had been culled because of infertility. Although death after foreign body penetration of the pericardium is usually caused by progressive fibrosing constrictive pericarditis and epicarditis, cardiac tamponade from perfora of the coronary artery also has been found.[20] Prognosis may be better for cattle in good body condition, with relatively normal appetite, able to ambulate, and less than 5 years old.[21]

Diaphragmatic Hernia

Diaphragmatic hernias are infrequently diagnosed in cattle. The most common clinical signs are recurrent rumen tympany (bloat), abdominal pain, diarrhea, dyspnea, anorexia, and weight loss.[22–25] Diaphragmatic defects have been diagnosed in young calves and adults.[26] Although traumatic reticuloperitonitis and congenital defects are thought to be the most common causes of diaphragmatic hernia in cattle, trauma (in calves from dystocia and in bulls from bull fights) and increased preparturient and parturient abdominal pressure should be considered.[27–30] The severity of clinical signs is related to the severity of visceral displacement into the thorax. Recently, the author treated a 4-month-old calf with peritoneopericardial hernia (**Fig. 2**). The calf suffered progressive dyspnea and was euthanatized during surgery because of the grave prognosis. Surgical correction has been described in cattle. A 10-cm by 8-cm defect in a 5-month-old heifer was closed using a nylon mesh implant via a right paramedian incision.[25] A 12-cm defect in an 18-month-old heifer was repaired via seventh rib resection and thoracotomy.[22] After closure of the diaphragmatic defect, pneumothorax was resolved by suctioning the remaining air from the thorax.

Pleuroscopy (Thoroscopy)

Thoroscopy is infrequently performed in cattle; however, the complete separation of the thorax by the mediastinum allows examination with creation of hemipneumothorax. Examination of the thorax and collection of diagnostic specimens (fine-needle aspirates, biopsy) is performed, and the carbon dioxide gas removed by suction. The author has performed thoroscopy for evaluation of pulmonary abscesses and pleuritis in several adult cattle. Widespread use of this technology is limited because specialized equipment is required and treatment of specific lesions is rare.

Surgical Approach to the Thorax

Surgery of the thorax of cattle is most commonly done for treatment of traumatic reticulopericarditis or reticulopleuritis;[18] however, thoracotomy has been reported for attempted treatment of stenosis of the pulmonary artery in a 10-month-old Holstein heifer.[31] Thoracotomy also has been used for treatment of pyothorax.[18,32] The surgical approach of choice is partial resection of the fifth or sixth rib to create a window into the cranioventral thorax. This surgery may be performed standing with local

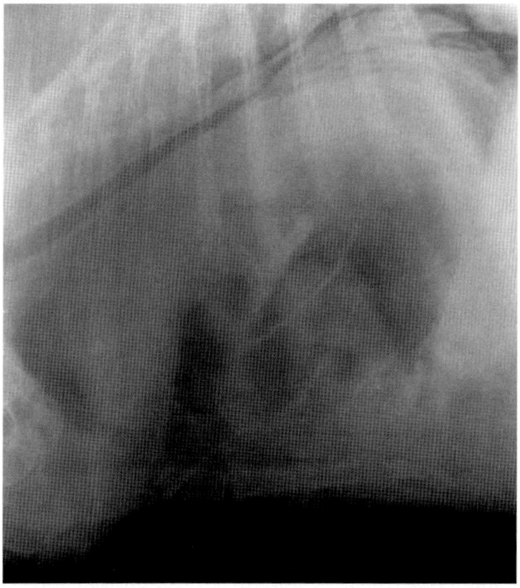

Fig. 2. Thoracic radiograph of a calf with exercise intolerance, open mouth breathing, weight loss, and a cough. Gas distension of bowel is evident in the region of the heart. Exploratory laparotomy revealed the presence of a peritoneopericardial hernia.

anesthesia, restrained on an inclined table with local anesthesia, or with the cow under general anesthesia. The author prefers to perform this surgery with the animal on an inclined table. Reticulopericarditis causes a progressive restrictive pericarditis resulting in limited ventricular filling and reduced cardiac output. Therefore, the cardiovascular side effects of general anesthesia may result in death. In one report of cattle having thoracotomy, fewer cattle on which surgery was performed under general anesthesia (one out of five cattle survived; three deaths were attributed to anesthetic complications) survived the procedure, compared with cattle having surgery performed on an inclined table (nine out of nine cattle survived).[18] The animal is placed on its right side on a tilt table at no more than a 45 degree angle.[33] Alternatively, a right thoracotomy may be performed.[18] The left (or right) front limb is pulled forward as far as possible and the fifth rib resected. An area extending from the sternum to the middle region of the thorax is clipped and prepared for aseptic surgery. The fifth or sixth rib is identified by counting forward from the last rib, and 2% lidocaine infused in a line block along the rib. Additional lidocaine is infused into the cranial and caudal intercostal spaces proximal and distal to the proposed surgery site. A linear incision is made along the fifth rib extending from the costochondral junction (at the level of the elbow) dorsally for approximately 15 cm. The lateral periosteum of the rib is incised and the periosteum elevated for the circumference of the rib. Obstetric wire is passed around the rib at the proximal and distal aspects of the incision. This portion of the rib is transected and removed. Then, the medial periosteum and parietal pleura are incised to expose the cranioventral thorax. Often with pericarditis the pericardium is adhered to the pleura. If the pericardium is not adhered to the pleura, the pericardial sac should be isolated from the pleural cavity before being opened. One author recommends decompression of the pericardial sac before pericardiotomy to avoid sudden decompression of the pericardium and cardiac arrest.[21] The pericardial sac is entered and drained. If the wire or foreign body can be found, it is removed. Often the foreign body has returned to the reticulum after penetrating the thorax. In the author's experience, laparotomy and rumenotomy causes excessive stress on affected cattle and may contribute to the demise of the animal. The author prefers to place a magnet into the reticulum until the survival of the patient has been determined. Alternatively, an instrument for removal of metallic foreign bodies has been developed and is useful for removal of those foreign bodies that can be attracted to a magnet.[34] The pericardium is marsupialized to the thoracic wall and skin using interrupted sutures (#3 braunamide, #2 PDS, for example) and the pericardial sac is lavaged with isotonic saline. Belt loop sutures are placed in the skin along the cranial and caudal margins of the incision, a stent bandage is placed over the wound, and umbilical tape is threaded through the belt loop sutures in a boot lace pattern to secure the bandage in place. Daily wound care involves lavage of the pericardial sac until the wound is closed. Alternatively, the pericardium and pleura may be closed in one layer; then the intercostal muscles and skin are closed individually. An indwelling drain may be placed into the pericardial sac before closure.

A similar approach is made for septic pleuritis or pulmonary abscess without entry into the pericardial sac, but the sixth or seventh rib is resected. After debridement and thorough lavage of the hemithorax has been performed, a drainage tube may be placed into the hemithorax through an adjacent stab incision and the thoracotomy wound closed primarily. The pleura, periosteum, and intercostal muscles are closed in one layer (interrupted or continuous pattern, #1 PDS), the muscles overlying the thoracic wall (latissimus dorsi, seratus ventralis thoracis, superficial pectoral, external abdominal oblique) are closed in one layer (interrupted or continuous pattern, #1 PDS), and the skin is closed routinely. The air remaining in the thorax is removed via the drainage tube and a Heimlich valve placed on the open end of the tube. Use of a Heimlich valve (one-way valve) allows continued drainage without compromise of thoracic pressure. A convenient way to construct a one-way valve is to attach a 15-cm long, 1.25-cm diameter Penrose drain onto the end of the chest tube. When the inner surface of the drain is wet, the sides of the Penrose drain will collapse on itself and provide a sufficient seal for the tube.

Surgery of the thorax is challenging under field conditions. A thorough risk-benefit analysis must be done to determine if the outcome justifies the cost of treatment and these must be taken in context with the prognosis.

REFERENCES

1. Callan RI, McGuirk SM, Step DL. Assessment of the cardiovascular and lymphatic systems. Vet Clin North Am Food Anim Pract 1992;8:257–70.
2. Pringle JK. Assessment of the ruminant respiratory system. Vet Clin North Am Food Anim Pract 1992;8:233–42.
3. Pringle JK. Ancillary testing for the ruminant respiratory system. Vet Clin North Am Food Anim Pract 1992;8:243–56.
4. Step DL, McGuirk SM, Callan RJ. Ancillary tests of the cardiovascular and lymphatic systems. Vet Clin North Am Food Anim Pract 1992;8:271–84.
5. Stober VM, Baackman W. Testing of a new instrument for the inspection of the oropharyngeal cavity and the entrance of the larynx in cattle. Dtsch Tierarztl Wochenschr 1978;85:189–272.
6. Tyler JW, Angel KL, Moll HD, et al. Something old, something new: thoracic acoustic percussion in cattle. J Am Vet Med Assoc 1990;197:52–7.
7. Anderson DE, DeBowes RM, Gaughan EM, et al. Endoscopic evaluation of the nasopharynx, pharynx, and larynx of Jersey cows. Am J Vet Res 1994;55:901–4.

8. Anderson DE, Gaughan EM, DeBowes RM, et al. Effects of chemical restraint on the endoscopic appearance of laryngeal and pharyngeal anatomy and sensation in adult cattle. Am J Vet Res 1994;55:1196–200.
9. Braun U, Fohn I, Pusterla N. Ultrasonographic examination of the ventral neck region in cows. Am J Vet Res 1994;55:14–21.
10. Braun U, Sicher D, Pusterla N. Ultrasonography of the lungs, pleura, and mediastinum in healthy cows. Am J Vet Res 1996;57:432–8.
11. Reef VB, Boy MG, Reid CF, et al. Comparison between diagnostic ultrasonography and radiography in the evaluation of horses and cattle with thoracic disease: 56 cases (1984–1985). J Am Vet Med Assoc 1991;198:2112–8.
12. Fingland RB, Rings DM, Vestweber JC. The etiology and surgical treatment of tracheal collapse in calves. Vet Surg 1990;19:371–9.
13. Vestweber JG, Leipold HW. Tracheal collapse in three calves. J Am Vet Assoc 1984;184:735–6.
14. Korney FD. Tracheal prosthesis in a calf. J Am Vet Med Assoc 1975;167:463–4.
15. Rings DM. Tracheal collapse. Vet Clin North Am Food Anim Pract 1995;11:171–6.
16. Ramakrishna O, Rao NY, Bose AS. Tracheal anastomosis in a heifer. J Am Vet Med Assoc 1980;177:547–8.
17. Braun U, Estermann U, Feige K, et al. Percutaneous lung biopsy in cattle. J Am Vet Med Assoc 1999;215:679–81.
18. Ducharme NG, Fubini SL, Renhun We, et al. Thoracotomy in adult dairy cattle: 14 cases (1979–1991). J Am Vet Med Assoc 1992;200:86–90.
19. McLennan MW, McGowan MR. Pyothorax in a Friesian bull. Aust Vet J 1995;72: 115–6.
20. Awadhiya RP, Kolte GN, Vegad JL. Cardiac tamponade: a fatal complication of traumatic reticulitis in cattle. Vet Rec 1974;95:260–2.
21. Noordsy JL. Rumenotomy, fistulation, cannulation, and pericardiotomy in cattle. In: Noordsy JL, Ames KN, editors. Food animal surgery. 4th edition. Yardley (PA): Veterinary Learning System; 2006. p. 111–26.
22. DeMoor A, Verschooten F, Desmet P. Thoracic repair of a diaphragmatic hernia in a heifer. Vet Rec 1969;85:87–8.
23. Done SH, Drew RA. Aperture in the diaphragm with protrusion of abnormal liver tissue: a report of three cases in the ox. Br Vet J 1972;128:553–9.
24. Hesselink JW. [Rupture in the diaphragm of a cow]. Tijdschr Diergeneeskd 1989; 114:1109–11 [in Dutch].
25. Troutt HF, Fessler JF, Page EH, et al. Diaphragmatic defects in cattle. J Am Vet Med Assoc 1967;151:1421–9.
26. Noordsy JL. Hernias and umbilical masses. In: Noordsy JL, editor. Food animal surgery. Lenexa (KS): Veterinary Medicine Publishing Company; 1989. p. 87–102.
27. Deore PA, Jahagirdar SS. Incidence of diaphragmatic hernia in cattle and buffaloes: case record of 16 cases. Indian Vet J 1971;48:1172–6.
28. Dhablania De, Tyagia RPS, Nigam JM. A study on diaphragmatic hernia in bovines. Indian Vet J 1971;48:91–8.
29. Homey FD, Cote J. Congenital diaphragmatic hernia in a calf. Can Vet J 1961;2: 422–4.
30. Hutchins DR, Blood DC, Hyne R. Residual defects in stomach motility after traumatic reticuloperitonitis of cattle: pyloric obstruction, diaphragmatic hernia, and indigestion due to reticular adhesions. Aust Vet J 1957;33:77–82.
31. Shiroya K, Saitoh Y, Muto M, et al. Crossed fat embolism in a cow with tetrology of fallot. J Vet Med Sci 1994;56:969–71.

32. St-Jean G, Smeak DD, Hubbell JAE, et al. Resolution of pyothorax in a white tailed deer by thoracotomy, tube drainage and lavage. Can Vet J 1990;31: 110–2.
33. Rings DM. Surgical treatment of pleuritis and pericarditis. Vet Clin North Am Food Anim Pract 1995;11:177–82.
34. Hekmati P, Bakshodeh GA, Poulsen JSD. Traumatic reticulitis, the comet naso reticular instrument for withdrawal of foreign bodies from the reticulum of cattle. Nord Vet Med 1985;37:338–48.

Physiologic Mastectomy via Flank Laparotomy

Andrew J. Allen, DVM*, George M. Barrington, DVM, PhD,
Steve M. Parish, DVM

KEYWORDS

• Mastectomy • Gangrenous mastitis • Mastitis
• Mammary gland • Physiologic mastectomy

INDICATIONS FOR USE

The external pudendal arteries provide the primary blood supply to the mammary glands, with a minor contribution provided by the ventral perineal arteries (**Fig. 1**). After emerging from the inguinal ring, the external pudendal artery branches to form the cranial mammary and caudal mammary arteries. Physiologic mastectomy (mastatrophy) involves reduction of the vascular supply to the mammary gland provided by the external pudendal artery, which causes tissue atrophy and possibly decreased systemic absorption of toxins liberated by affected glands. Indications include chronic suppurative mastitis, gangrenous mastitis, and chronic, severe mastitis associated with organisms that liberate endotoxin (eg, *Escherichia coli*, *Klebsiella* spp) or exotoxin (eg, *Staphylococcus* spp). Physiologic mastectomy via flank laparotomy is strictly a salvage procedure. Improved survival rates and decreased convalescence time have been reported with similar mammary vessel ligation procedures.[1] The procedure can be performed rapidly and is significantly less complicated and traumatic than a complete or hemi-mastectomy.

ANESTHESIA AND SURGICAL PREPARATION

The procedure is performed with the animal standing. The surgical approach is typically via the side ipsilateral to the mastitic or affected gland; however, it can be performed from the contralateral side if adhesions from previous surgeries are present. The paralumbar fossa is clipped and a routine surgical preparation is performed. Local anesthesia is administered in a routine manner using an "inverted L," distal parvertebral, or line block.

Department of Veterinary Clinical Sciences, Washington State University, PO Box 647060, Pullman, WA 99164-7060, USA
* Corresponding author.
E-mail address: aja@vetmed.wsu.edu (A.J. Allen).

Vet Clin Food Anim 24 (2008) 511–516
doi:10.1016/j.cvfa.2008.06.006 vetfood.theclinics.com
0749-0720/08/$ – see front matter © 2008 Elsevier Inc. All rights reserved.

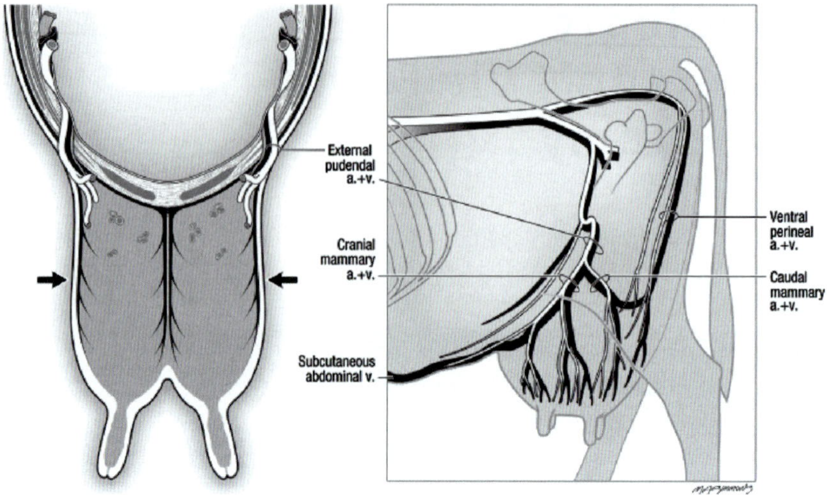

Fig. 1. Blood supply to the bovine mammary gland.

SURGICAL TECHNIQUE

An approximately 20-cm incision is made in the mid-paralumbar fossa beginning approximately 8 cm ventral to the lumbar transverse processes. Sharp dissection through all muscle layers or a grid approach can be used, depending on the surgeon's preference. A brief exploration of abdominal structures is suggested to rule out other conditions that may affect prognosis.

The external pudendal artery is a branch of the pudendoepigastric trunk, which in turn is a branch of the internal iliac artery. The external pudendal artery and vein are located by palpating along the internal abdominal wall caudal to the incision as they enter the internal inguinal ring (approximately 10 cm ventral and lateral to the pubic symphysis). The pulse and size of the artery (1–2 cm diameter) are easily recognized as the vessel penetrates the internal inguinal ring exiting the abdominal cavity (**Fig. 2**). The external pudendal artery and vein are isolated immediately proximal to the internal inguinal ring via blunt dissection to separate the vessels from the peritoneal

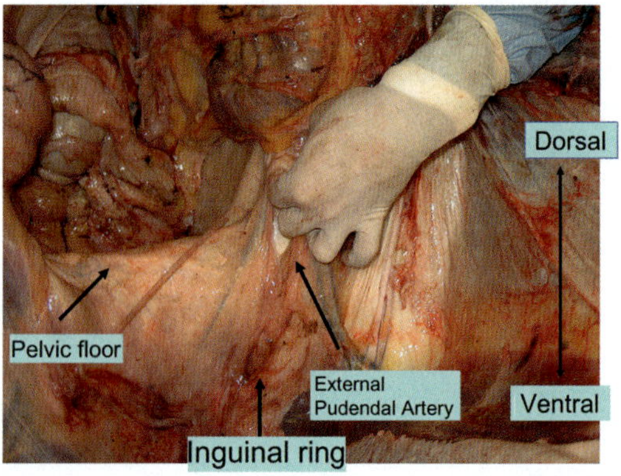

Fig. 2. Find the external pudendal artery as it transverses through the inguinal ring.

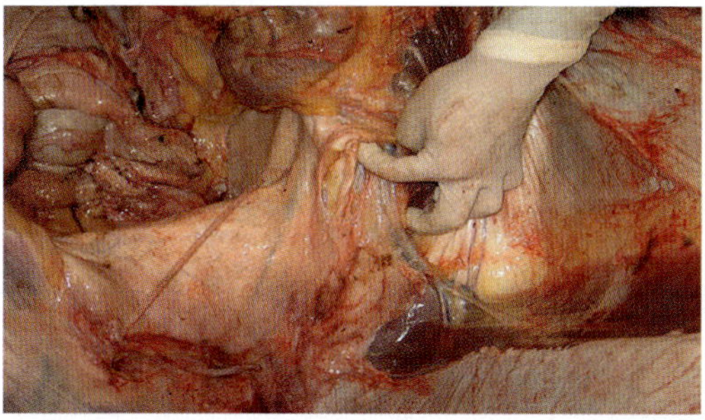

Fig. 3. Bluntly dissect the vessels from the body wall with tips of fingers and thumb.

membrane, fat, and connective tissue (**Fig. 3**). It is important to free the vessels from most of the surrounding connective tissue to allow for proper ligation. Adequate dissection is achieved when the operator can insert two fingers completely around the vessels (**Fig. 4**). Ligation can be achieved using any large, nonabsorbable suture material. We have found that the use of a sterilized cable tie in place of suture material greatly aids in the speed and ease of ligation (**Figs. 5–7**).

Once the cable tie is placed, the artery distal is palpated to detect any remnant pulse. If a pulse is present, the tie is further tightened. Once ligation is deemed successful, the tie can be trimmed short or left untrimmed, and the abdomen is closed in a routine manner. In concurrence with other authors,[2,3] we consider the contribution of the ventral perineal artery and vein to be insignificant and do not ligate it in this procedure.

If a cow is systemically compromised, postoperative antibiotics and anti-inflammatory drugs can be administered. Cases of chronic, suppurative mastitis may benefit from drainage of the quarter by concurrent teat amputation. In most

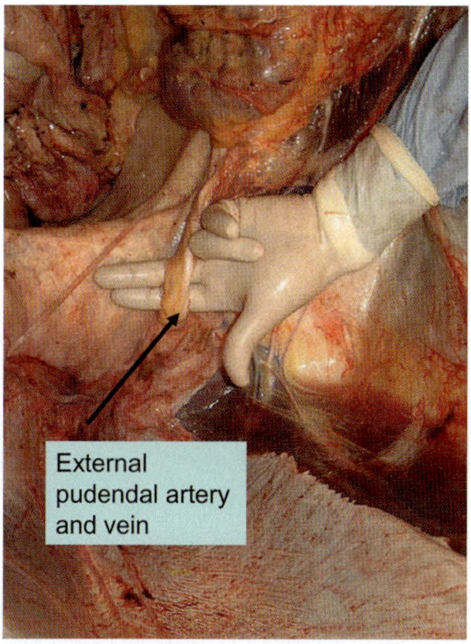

Fig. 4. Dissect the vessels until you can get two fingers between the vessels and the body wall.

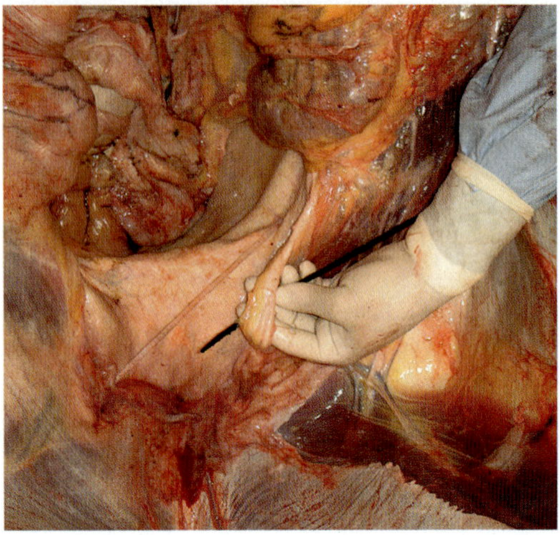

Fig. 5. Insert cable tie under vessels.

cases, the noticeable atrophy of the gland does not occur for 6 to 8 weeks after surgery. Frequently, we observe resumption of eating within 1 to 2 days after surgery in animals that were anorectic preoperatively.

DISCUSSION

Other techniques for physical or physiologic mastectomy in the cow have been described, including ligation of the external pudendal artery via a transvaginal approach or an external inguinal approach and a complete mastectomy.[1–4] Advantages of the physiologic mastectomy procedure described herein include decreased operative time, a more simplified and standard approach, and completion of the procedure using local anesthesia while the animal is standing. Disadvantages include the need to enter the abdominal cavity, the blind approach, and occlusion of the blood supply to an entire half of the gland. The procedure is a simple yet effective alternative to radical mastectomy for cases of unresponsive mastitis in genetically valuable or otherwise valued cattle. The procedure also may be an effective salvage option in decreasing mortality and convalescence with cattle that suffer severe gangrenous or toxin-producing mastitis and would typically be euthanized.

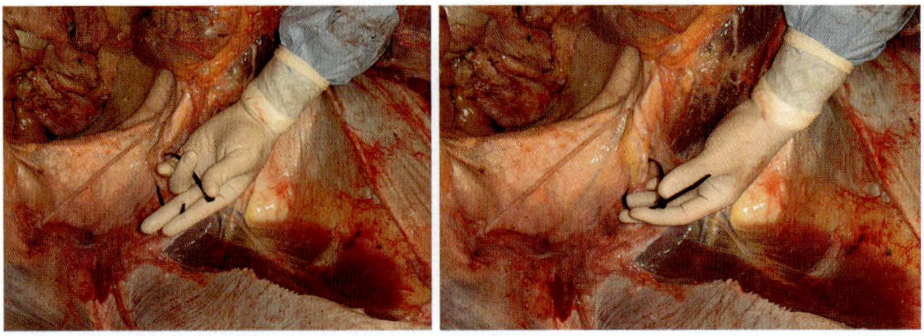

Fig. 6. Insert cable tie into ratchet case and tighten.

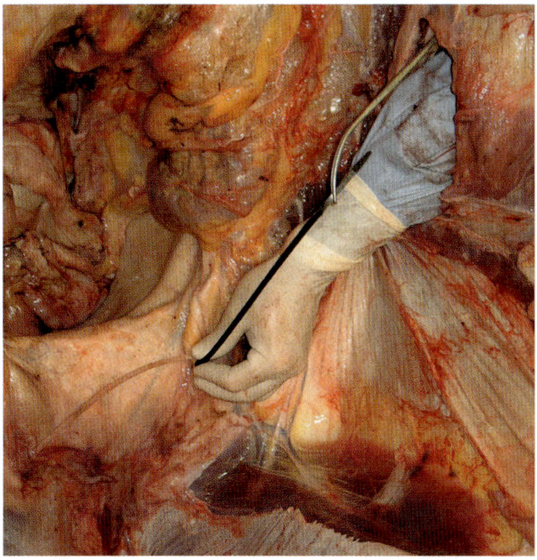

Fig. 7. Long-handled carmalt forceps can assist in tightening the cable tie.

The long-term effects of physiologic mastectomy are less well described and are likely to depend on the severity and etiology of the original mastitic episode. Anecdotal evidence in beef cattle suggests a good prognosis for the life of the cow and her ability to raise a calf on the functional half of the original mammary tissue. The procedure in dairy cattle is clearly recommended for salvage purposes and to prolong the life of genetically valuable individuals because milk production is affected significantly. In humans, incomplete ligation can result in the formation of thrombi.[5] On limited occasions, we have observed thrombosis of the external pudendal artery and suspected the cause to be related to an incomplete ligation (**Fig. 8**). Finally, one could assume an increased risk for aneurysm formation proximal to the ligature; however, this complication has not been observed to date.

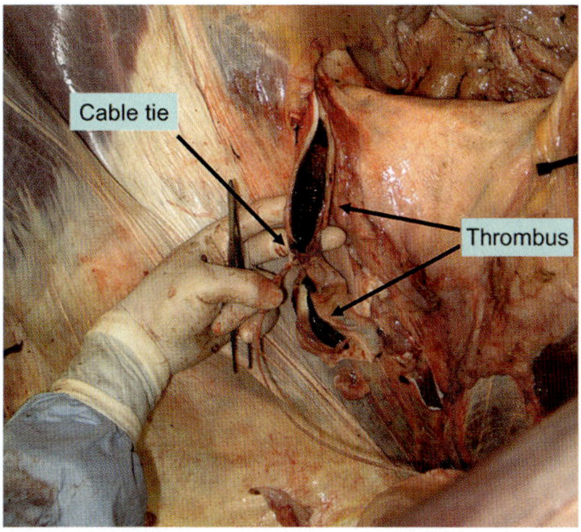

Fig. 8. Thrombosed vessel opened with cable tie in the center.

REFERENCES

1. Brewer RL. Mammary vessel ligation for gangrenous mastitis. J Am Vet Med Assoc 1963;143:44–5.
2. El-Maghraby HM. Comparison of two surgical techniques for mastectomy of goats. Small Rumin Res 2001;40(3):215–21.
3. Noordsy JL. Food animal surgery. Lenexa (KS): Veterinary Medicine Publishing Company; 1989. p. 238–43.
4. Cable CS, Peery K, Fubini SL. Radical mastectomy in 20 ruminants. Vet Surg 2004;33(3):263–6.
5. Oneglia C, Muneretto C, Rusconi C. Transesophageal investigation of surgically ligated left atrial appendage. Echocardiography 2004;21(7):617–9.

Bovine Surgery of the Skin

Matt D. Miesner, DVM, MS

KEYWORDS

• Bovine • Skin • Dermis • Repair • Cosmetic • Healing

Within just the past decade, scientific evidence regarding bovine pain and distress responses to surgical stimuli has grown immensely. Although most of the work to date is subjective in nature, objective measures of painful responses are being applied more commonly to address animal welfare concerns. It is important to be cognizant of these findings. Efforts should be made to incorporate animal comfort and welfare in surgical decision-making processes to enhance productivity as a whole.

GENERAL SKIN WOUND HEALING

The skin provides a vital protective barrier to the body. Mechanisms to repair breeches of that barrier during wounding follow a predictable and efficient pattern in mammalian species. The process is often simplified to grasp the concept of the repair process, but in actuality it involves a complex interaction of cells, fluid and protein constituents, and chemical mediators. The first general concept of wound healing is the phases of repair that include inflammation, followed by proliferation, and finally, remodeling. One must first recognize that these phases involve significant time frame overlap during transition. In addition, each primary phase can be divided into subsets with unique mechanisms of repair. Primary surgical closure rapidly concentrates the healing process with more overlap between phases. Second intension healing results in an exaggerated length of time to closure, depending on the size of the wound and the complications arising during the healing process. The reader is referred to other sources for detailed information on wound healing.[1] For a summary of the stages of wound healing relevant to this text, refer to **Fig. 1** and **Table 1**.

Managing Skin Wounds

Complications leading to delays in the healing process often occur. A basic understanding of wound healing can aid in successful wound management. Nonhealing cutaneous wounds may be due to foreign material (metal, organic debris, and so forth) within the wound, periosteitis, or bone sequestrum deep to the wound. Periosteitis should be considered in the presence of chronic draining tracks even when severing

Department of Clinical Sciences, College of Veterinary Medicine, Kansas State University, 1800 Dennison Avenue, Manhattan, KS 66506, USA
E-mail address: mmiesner@vet.k-state.edu

Vet Clin Food Anim 24 (2008) 517–526
doi:10.1016/j.cvfa.2008.06.001 vetfood.theclinics.com
0749-0720/08/$ – see front matter © 2008 Elsevier Inc. All rights reserved.

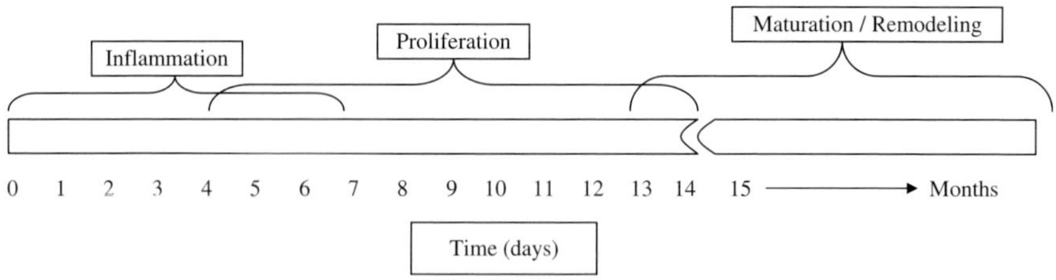

Fig. 1. Phases of wound healing and general time frame of each phase. Epithelialization, a division of proliferation, can be seen histologically at wound edges within the first days of injury.

the skin was not in the history. Blunt trauma in bony areas with little soft tissue protection and crush injury, as might be the case with calving chain trauma, can present in this manner. Nearly all traumatic wounds in bovine practice will be plagued with gross contamination by the time of recognition. It is not uncommon to begin with a wound that is caked with mud, manure, straw, or gravel. A significant delay between the time the wound occurred and injury is recognized is also a common woe, which would therefore suggest that the wound will either have to heal by second intention or delayed primary closure. A third option commonly involves initial primary skin closure to draw the wound periphery "closer" together, providing initial protection over a wound ultimately destined to heal by second intention. The latter option is reasonable, provided drainage from the deep portions of the wound is adequate.

The first order of business is to focus on controlling the inflammatory process, reducing edema, assisting with wound debridement, and treating infection. Regarding inflammation, the goal should be to modulate the inflammatory process and not block it entirely. The aim should be to control an exaggerated systemic inflammatory response while not suppressing neutrophil migration and function within the wound as a normal part of the healing process. Glucocorticoids have been shown to downregulate L-selectin binding, necessary for migration of neutrophils from capillary endothelium, and to delay necessary neutrophil apoptosis for macrophage phagocytosis and sequential functions in the healing process.[2,3] Nonsteroidal anti-inflammatory drugs (NSAIDS) may modulate inflammation more effectively without deleterious effects on cellular function.[4] The clinical debate about the use of steroidal versus nonsteroidal drugs or combinations in the face of infection is ongoing. Edema within a wound can be treated with compression wraps when possible, and hydrotherapy, increasing perfusion and debriding the wound.

Physical debridement of the wound should be undertaken with initial assessment, noting clinical characteristics, severity, structures involved, and estimating the duration. Gentle scrubbing of the wound initially with antiseptics will remove large debris. If povidone iodine is used for scrub/lavage, it should be a dilute solution (~ %), because "free" iodine in solution is the basis for antimicrobial activity. The amount of free iodine in a solution increases as the concentration decreases. Wound lavage with dilute antiseptic solution can then be used. The author prefers lavage with an 18-gauge needle and syringe to provide targeted focal hydro pressure and debridement.

Infection should initially be treated empirically using broad-spectrum systemic antibiotics and topical antiseptic therapy. The wound should be reassessed frequently and culture and sensitivity should guide antibiotic therapy when unresolved infection appears to be complicating the healing process. Intravenous regional antibiotic infusion could be argued in cases of distal limb wounds, with the thought that higher concentrations of drug in the area of interest could be achieved. The counterargument

Table 1
Basic summary of phase designations, approximate timing, and general physiology during healing of an uncomplicated wound

Healing Phase (Clinical Characteristics)	Time	Intraphase Designations	Description
Inflammation (edema, exudate, blood clot, scab)	At time of injury	Capillary permeability changes	Initial serotonin-mediated vasoconstriction in the first 5 to 10 minutes after injury Histamine-mediated vasodilatation follows with increased vascular permeability, flooding wound with blood constituents for hemostasis and cell recruitment signals for later phases of repair.
		Exudation: fibrin and glycoprotein deposition	Forms bridgework for cellular migration in later phases Initial weak cell matrix to be replaced by granulation tissue during proliferative phase
	1 to 6 days post injury	Destruction	Leukocyte (neutrophil) chemotaxis Lysosomal enzyme digestion of debris and wound contaminants and signal monocyte migration to wound Collagenase degradation of matrix
		Debridement	Macrophages further debride wound of debris and signal for cell recruitment of cells and constituents for proliferative phase.
Proliferation (granulation tissue)	3 to 14 days post injury	Epithelialization	Begins within the first couple of days after injury at the periphery of wound (microscopically), and is set to migrate across bridge formed by cellular counterparts during proliferative phase Grossly evident at periphery of wound at about 2 weeks
		Fibroplasia	Fibroblast proliferation for collagen, proteoglycans, and extracellular matrix formation for delivery of necessary constituents of cell growth
		Angiogenesis	Intricate series of steps to form new blood vessels traversing the wound
Maturation/ remodeling (scar tissue)	~14 days onward	Contraction	Tightening of healed wound through myofibroblast tensioning on microfilaments in the extracellular matrix Fibroblast degradation of matrix, thus pulling edges of wound closer together
		Remodeling	Balancing collagen synthesis and catabolism within wound

would be that the antibiotics that are safe and legal to use in this manner, namely B-lactams, have time above minimum inhibitory concentration-dependent mechanisms of action, not concentration dependent.[5] On the other hand, intravenous regional antibiotic perfusion should provide more rapid distribution of the dose within the area of concern.[6]

Primary Closure of Contaminated Wounds

Primary skin closure over a contaminated wound is a reasonable decision provided adequate drainage from the deep portions of the wound is provided. Primary partial closure of gaping wounds will benefit the healing process later on by concentrating the time frame and distance during the proliferative stages and by decreasing the degree of wound contraction during remodeling. Portions of the wound should remain open to provide a portal for wound lavage and discharge of the products of inflammation. Consideration should be given to the orientation of the blood supply to the affected area in regard to the placement and type of tension-relieving suture patterns (**Fig. 2**). Vertical mattress sutures (with and without stents) and near-far-far-near suture

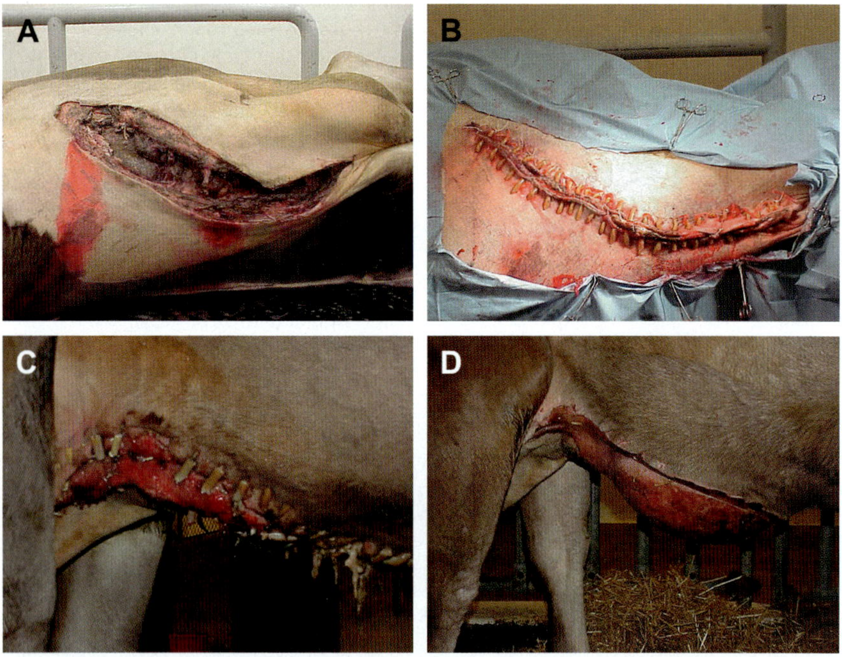

Fig. 2. (*A*) Large contaminated ventral abdominal wound in a pregnant Brown Swiss heifer. The laceration begins adjacent to the brisket cranially and ends caudally, just shy of the subcutaneous abdominal (milk) vein near the udder. Only peritoneum prevents entry into the abdominal cavity. (*B*) The wound was cleaned and superficially debrided before closure with # 3 Braunamid (double strands) with multiple vertical mattress sutures using simplex tubing as stents. (*C*) Approximately 2.5 weeks post–wound closure. Note wound proliferation and expelled exudate, and tension on stents in skin. (*D*) Approximately 6 weeks post–wound closure. Healthy granulation bed traversing wound, with skin proliferation at periphery. Bulge in granulation due to progressing, late, third trimester pregnancy. A flank cesarean section was performed to remove the calf, followed by debridement and closure of the wound 1 week later. Complete healing noted 2 months after delayed primary closure of wound.

patterns are favored whenever possible to relieve tension, preserve collateral blood supply and, in cases of contaminated wounds, provide intermittent gaps for escaping exudate.

SURGICAL DEHORNING OF CATTLE

Surgical Dehorning Considerations

Surgical dehorning of cattle, often referred to as cosmetic dehorning, is discussed in this article. For a lengthier description regarding surgical dehorning, the reader is directed to the March 1995 issue of this text.[7] Many methods of dehorning cattle exist, from basic cautery in young cattle, to straightforward removal in older cattle using various techniques. Closure of the resulting wound would constitute surgical dehorning regardless of the desired cosmetic outcome. Ethical decisions need to be made on an individual basis when goals are purely cosmetic or when removing scurs in designated polled animals. One should recognize that a desirable cosmetic appearance can be achieved with many of the more simplistic methods of dehorning; however, surgical dehorning has some added advantages (see later discussion). Dehorning or disbudding young calves should be undertaken whenever possible to reduce animal stress and chances of complications. The author supports local anesthesia regardless of the age of the animal or the dehorning method used.

Dehorning cattle is advocated for improving cattle and worker safety, facilitating handling, feeding efficiently at allotted bunk spaces, and improving carcass quality and animal health with less muscle bruising. Surgical dehorning reduces healing time, provides accurate hemostasis, and eliminates an open wound that may communicate with the frontal sinus. Veterinary intervention for the surgical procedure and presence on the farm, ranch, or feed yard has its own advantages from a herd health standpoint. Eliminating an open wound prevents fly strike and greatly reduces the chance of soft tissue infection with good surgical technique. Theoretically, the risk for sinusitis should also be reduced because an open sinus will not be continually exposed to environmental contaminants and precautions are taken to facilitate drainage (see later discussion).

Surgical Procedure

The animal should be adequately restrained in a squeeze chute and head catch that allows access to both horns. Additional head restraint is necessary and can be accomplished with the use of halters and lead ropes, tying the lead closely to one side and then the other. Squeeze chutes with a mechanical head restraint apparatus are an added benefit when available and prevent the need to reposition the patient between sides. Sedation with low doses of intravenous xylazine (0.01 mg/kg to 0.04 mg/kg) may be adequate for standing anesthesia and a cooperative patient. The clinician should start with the lower end of the dosing spectrum and titrate as needed. Alternatively, a combination of butorphanol (0.01 mg/kg), xylazine (0.02 mg/kg), and ketamine (0.04 mg/kg) intramuscular or subcutaneous has been used effectively with good results for standing sedation by the author and it provides additional analgesia.

A wide surgical field should be clipped around each horn, across the forehead, and behind the pole. A surgical prep with povidone iodine or chlorhexidine and isopropyl alcohol should be performed. Local anesthesia with 2% lidocaine can then be performed, beginning at the location of the cornual nerve at the frontal crest of the skull (**Fig. 3**), then extending the block subcutaneously around each horn as a ring block. The initial focal block of the cornual nerve provides most of the analgesia;

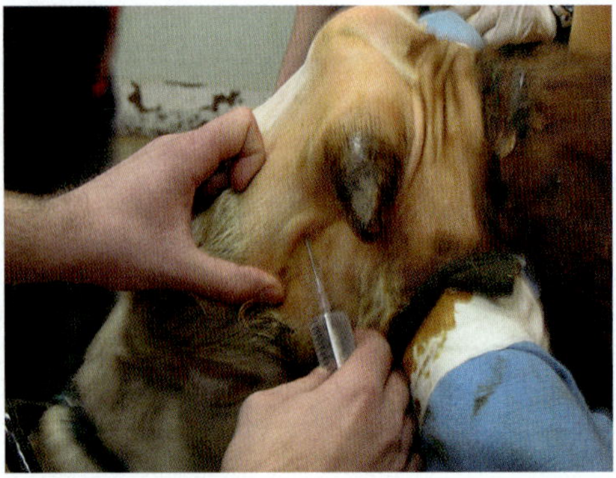

Fig. 3. Anesthetizing the cornual nerve at the facial crest. The block is then continued as a ring block around the horn. Note the clipped surgical field and clean towels covering the ears.

however, branches of the cranial cervical nerves may provide some sensory input to the caudal horn, hence the reasoning behind the ring block. A second surgical prep after local anesthesia is advisable. The ears should be retracted away from the surgical field, or alternatively, wrapped with clean towels or drape material. The head should not be draped because evaluation of symmetry will need to be monitored during surgery.

A full-thickness skin incision, beginning near the pole and extending in an elliptic fashion around the base and ending ventral to the horn, should be made. An attempt should be made to make a clean incision with two full-thickness passes on the anterior and posterior sides of the horn. The scalpel blade should be maintained at a perpendicular angle to the skin. To prevent partial horn regrowth (scurs), the corium of the horn should be avoided by approximately 0.75 to 1 cm at the widest part of the ellipse. The author initially avoids incising much subcutaneous tissue at

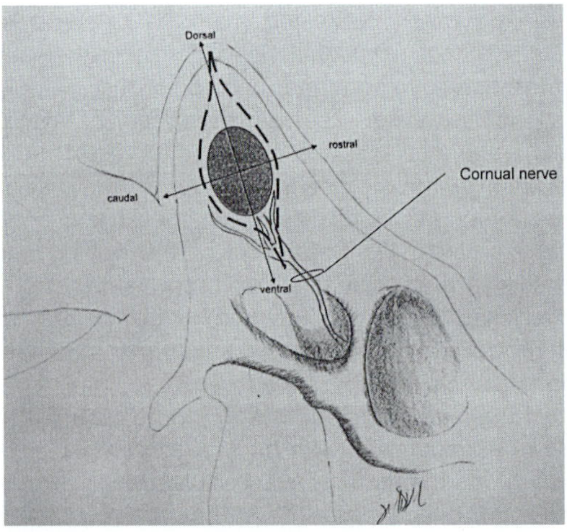

Fig. 4. Orientation of the elliptic incision (*dashed line*) around the horn for removal. (*Courtesy of* Matt Miesner, DVM, MS, Manhattan, KS.)

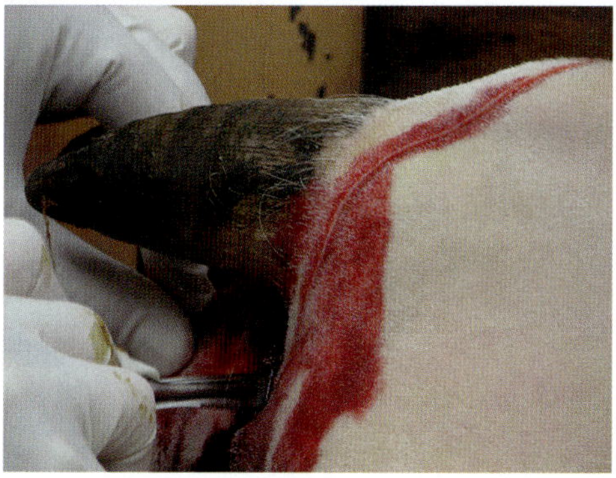

Fig. 5. Orientation of the anterior incision when viewed from the front.

the ventral apex of the ellipse to prevent cutting the cornual artery. Care should be taken to orient the incision parallel to the long axis of the horn (**Figs. 4–6**). Using a scalpel, the skin to be removed should be undermined up to the base of the horn and the skin to be preserved should be undermined 1 to 2 cm from the cut edges, which allows easy horn access while preventing trauma to the skin to be sutured during horn removal. One should not spend a great deal of time searching for hemorrhaging vessels at this point.

Removing the horn and bone followed by hemostasis are the next steps. Barnes dehorners are effective for removing horn and bone and avoiding skin trauma when oriented parallel to the incision (**Fig. 7**). Obstetric wire can be used for removal of larger horns, being careful not to damage the preserved skin as the wire heats up during use (**Fig. 8**). Once the horn is removed, hemostasis should be commenced by isolating the cornual artery at the ventral base of the horn, then either ligating, twisting, or extracting the vessel. A method used by the author for hemostasis when using obstetric wire is to stop sawing at the ventral margin of the incision after the bone of the horn is cut. One should grasp the horn, pulling down and twisting in one direction until the cornual artery is extracted. After horn removal and hemostasis, the Barnes dehorner, or bone chisel and mallet, can aid in controlled bone removal to shape the skull and remove bone to facilitate skin closure. One should

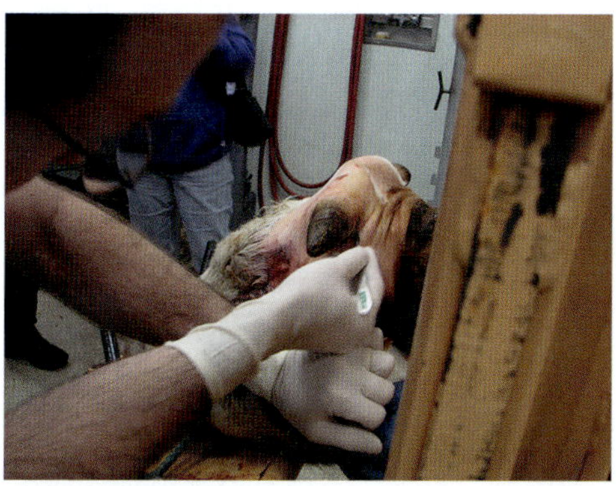

Fig. 6. It is important to reduce the skin folds when incising the posterior skin, to prevent inadvertently removing excessive skin.

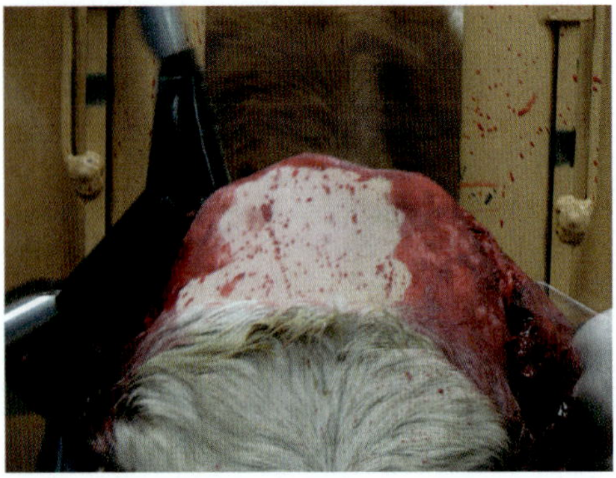

Fig. 7. The Barnes dehorner oriented parallel to the long axis of the incision while removing horn and excess bone.

observe closely for bone fragments and fractures that could serve as a nidus for infection or sequestra after closure. Any loose fragments should be removed before closure. If the frontal sinus was opened during surgery, as is usually the case, debris should be prevented from entering the sinus cavity. Occasionally, a thin periosteal membrane lining the sinus can be seen after horn removal. If the membrane remains once the desired amount of bone is removed, the author prefers to perforate the membrane to facilitate drainage through the sinus and prevent accumulation of inflammatory debris during healing.

Attempt to oppose the skin edges for closure, continuing to undermine anterior and posterior sharply until the skin edges can be opposed under little tension. More skin mobility and tension relief will arise from the posterior margin, but one must be cognizant and avoid traumatizing the auricular tissues. Once the skin edges can be opposed, the suture pattern is left to the discretion of the surgeon. Typically, a #2 or #3 nonabsorbable suture is selected for the single layer closure. A simple continuous suture pattern can be used when little tension exists and is rapid and cosmetic. A forward interlocking pattern is also quick to place and provides more tension relief. The author prefers an inverted cruciate pattern (**Fig. 9**) that is cosmetic, relieves tension,

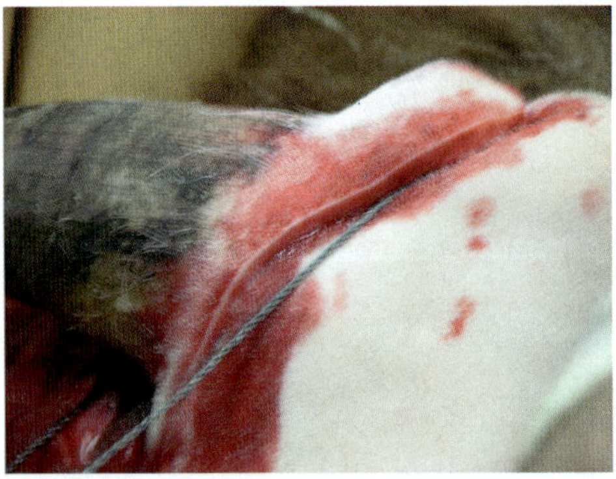

Fig. 8. Obstetric wire used to remove the horn. Caution must be used so as not to traumatize the skin to be preserved with the wire.

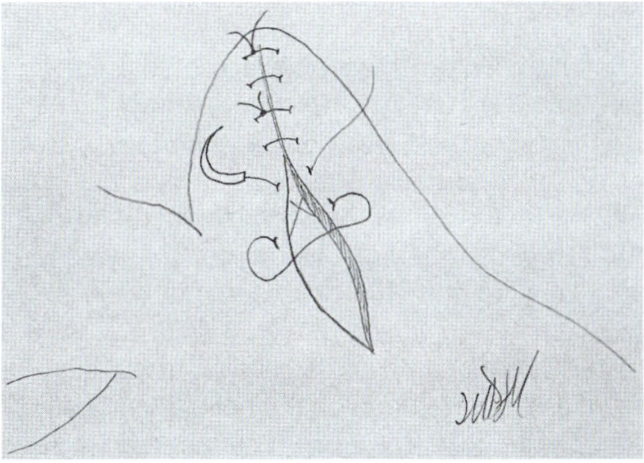

Fig. 9. Inverted cruciate pattern during skin closure. (*Courtesy of* Matt Miesner, DVM, MS, Manhattan, KS.)

preserves the ability to open part of the incision for drainage should infection arise, and prevents loss of the entire line should the animal break part of the suture during healing. Intradermal closure with #0 or #1 absorbable monofilament suture has been performed, but extra precaution and monitoring should be undertaken by the client during recovery to address the complications listed earlier (**Fig. 10**).

Once the opposite horn has been removed symmetric to the first side, the patient should be cleaned off thoroughly. A small amount of hemorrhage originating from the frontal sinus and draining from the nares is common and may be present for the first day after surgery. Applying topical wound ointments or sprays to the surgical site should be avoided if possible; nitrofurazone is now strictly forbidden for use in animals intended for food in the United States. When drugs, including those for sedation, antibiotics, and anti-inflammatory drugs, are used, meat- and milk-withholding times should be clearly stated. Sutures can be removed as early as 10 days postoperatively, but often, 2 weeks is recommended. The client should avoid placing the animal in situations where self-inflicted trauma and wound contamination may occur. In the author's experience, the first few hours after surgery, coinciding with the waning effects of the lidocaine, appear to be the most common time for the animal to rub on the incision. An itemized patient discharge form, describing postoperative care and potential complications of the procedure, facilitates client recognition and follow-up care, if needed.

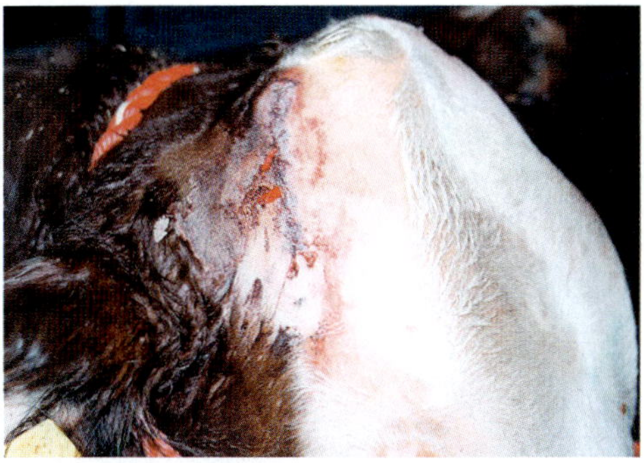

Fig. 10. Closure of a surgical dehorn using an intradermal suture pattern with #1 absorbable monofilament suture.

REFERENCES

1. Theoret CL. The pathophysiology of wound repair. Vet Clin North Am Equine Pract. Philadelphia:Saunders; 2005;21(1):1–13.
2. Weber PS, Madsen-Bouterse SA, Rosa GJ, et al. Analysis of the bovine neutrophil transcriptome during glucocorticoid treatment. Physiol Genomics 2006;28:97–112.
3. Weber PSD, Toelboell T, Chang LC, et al. Mechanisms of glucocorticoid-induced down-regulation of neutrophil L-selectin in cattle: evidence for effects at the gene-expression level and primarily on blood neutrophils. J Leukoc Biol 2005; 75:815–27.
4. Bednarek D, Szuster-Ciesielska A, Zdzisiñska B, et al. The effect of steroidal and non-steroidal anti-inflammatory drugs on the cellular immunity of calves with experimentally-induced local lung inflammation. Vet Immunol Immunopathol 1999;71(1): 1–15.
5. Fajt VR, Apley MD. Antimicrobial issues in bovine lameness. Vet Clin North Am Food Anim Pract. Piladelphia:Saunders; 2001;17(1):159–73.
6. Navarre CB, Zhang L, Sunkara G, et al. Ceftiofur distribution in plasma and joint fluid following regional limb injection in cattle. J Vet Pharmacol Ther 1999;22:13–9.
7. Hoffsis G. Surgical (cosmetic) dehorning in cattle. Vet Clin North Am Food Anim Pract. Piladelphia:Saunders; 1995;11(1):159–69.

Field Surgery of the Eye and Para-Orbital Tissues

Kara Schulz, DVM

KEYWORDS

• Ocular • Surgery • Eye • Bovine

Ocular disease and injury remain a common occurrence in cattle. In many instances medical management is sufficient for resolution and amelioration of clinical signs. In selected cases, surgical intervention is required. Fortunately, field surgery remains a viable option for most cases of bovine ocular disease. While the surgical techniques are not new, thorough physical examination, proper preparation of the patient, appropriate perioperative management, and good surgical technique will assure the best results possible.

OCULAR EXAMINATION

Diagnosis

A thoroughly performed systematic physical examination and ocular examination of the cow is vital to determining the correct diagnosis and extent of disease (**Fig. 1**). These examination findings will dictate the potential surgical options and associated prognosis for survival, return to productivity, and risk of subsequent condemnation at slaughter. Factors such as age, pregnancy status, and economic value influence the owner's decision regarding treatment.

Restraint

Proper restraint will allow for a thorough examination of the eye. For most cattle a chute with halter restraint is sufficient; however, mild sedation may be required in some cattle. Care must be taken in dosing sedation as to avoid recumbency in cattle and abortion in pregnant cows. Use of local anesthesia (eg, Lidocaine HCl) to induce regional anesthesia of the eye by sensory and motor blockade greatly facilitates examination and treatment.

Motor Blockade of Upper Eyelid

Motor blockade of the associated eyelid musculature and sensory blockade of corneal nerve endings can greatly enhance the ease of examination. Motor innervation to the upper eyelid musculature can be blocked via an auriculopalpebral nerve block. This is

Department of Clinical Sciences, College of Veterinary Medicine, Kansas State University, Manhattan, KS 66506, USA
E-mail address: kschulz@vet.ksu.edu

Vet Clin Food Anim 24 (2008) 527–534
doi:10.1016/j.cvfa.2008.07.003 vetfood.theclinics.com
0749-0720/08/$ – see front matter © 2008 Published by Elsevier Inc.

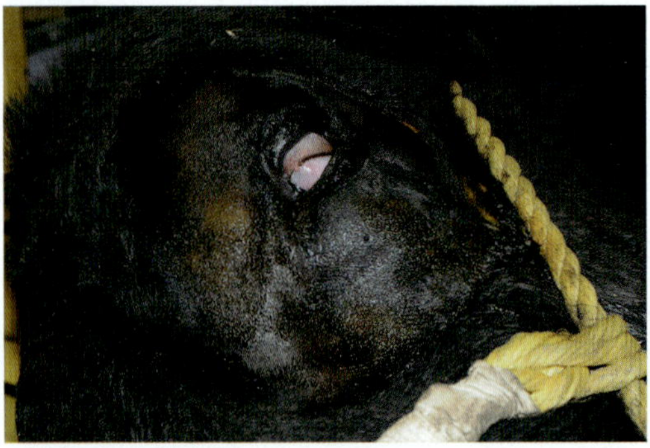

Fig. 1. Adult angus bull with panuveitis and corneal abscess secondary to trauma. (*Courtesy of* David Adams, Manhattan, KS and David E. Anderson, DVM, MS, Manhattan, KS.)

accomplished by infiltrating 5 mL to 6 mL of a 2% lidocaine solution into the subcutaneous tissue along the dorsal aspect of the zygomatic arch roughly 5 cm to 6 cm caudal to the frontal process of the zygomatic bone (ie, caudal to the lateral canthus of eye).

Sensory Blockade of Cornea

Sensory blockade of the corneal surface will also aid in examination of the eye. Administering 3 to 5 drops of proparacaine (1%) ophthalmic solution topically to the corneal surface of the eye will reduce corneal sensation.

Examination

The extent of ocular examination will be dictated by the clinical signs present. Fluorescein stain can be used to detect the presence of corneal ulcers. Intraocular disease will require the use of an ophthalmoscope and topical instillation of drops to dilate the pupil. Any masses visible within the lid margins, third eyelid, conjunctiva, or sclera should be palpated with a gloved and lubricated finger to determine degree of infiltration into adjacent periorbital structures. The third eyelid can be grasped with an atraumatic forcep to facilitate exteriorization and examination of the base of the nictitating membrane.

PATIENT SURGICAL PREPARATION

Restraint

Proper restraint is essential for surgical manioulation of the eye and para-orbital tissues. Most bovine field surgeries can be performed with the patient standing in a chute or head catch, with the head securely restrained in a head catch with a halter or some type of head board restraint.

Surgical Site Preparation

Infection of the surgical site is one of the most common complications of ocular surgery done when done in field settings. Care must be taken to reduce the risk of contamination to the planned surgical site. The hair should be clipped, the skin disinfected with solutions such as betadine or chlorhexadine, the ear should be draped, and the lateral portion of the halter covered to decrease contamination to the surgical site. Saline rinse rather than alcohol should be used between the disinfectant scrubs to prevent irritation and damage to the cornea. An ophthalmic ointment should be placed on the cornea before aseptic preparation to further protect the cornea from damage in cases other than enucleation.

ANESTHESIA

Sedation

Appropriate sedation as described previously may be warranted in certain cattle. The author most often uses xylazine (0.05 mg/kg body weight intravenously or IV) and butorphenol (0.02 mg/kg IV) for standing restraint. Addition of dissociative doses of ketamine (0.1 mg/kg IV) aids in management of fractious patients and these three drugs in combination have been referred to as a "Ket-Stun" technique.

Local Anesthesia

Local anesthesia to the intended surgical site will assure comfort on the part of the cow undergoing the procedure, as well as ease in handling for the surgeon.

Nerve Blocks

The nerve blocks outlined below are described in several text books.[1–7] Reasons for choosing one block over the other should include the surgeon's comfort and skill at performing the blocks, the disease process present, and the knowledge of the risks associated with each block. While the Peterson eye block is considered more technically challenging, it is associated with less risk of trauma to the orbit with regards to penetration of the globe, hemorrhage, and damage to the optic nerve. However, there are risks of neurologic signs or death because of cardiopulmonary arrest if lidocaine is injected into the optic nerve meninges or nasal turbinates. The 4-point block is technically less challenging to perform and appears to yield better anesthesia of the periocular tissues. While there is risk of intrameningeal injection, the authors' clinical experience has shown it to be less of an issue than with the Peterson nerve block.

Auriculopalpebral Nerve Block

Surgical manipulation of the eye is facilitated by nerve blockade of the eyelids. Auriculopalpebral nerve block can be placed to reduce upper eyelid movement before performing a Peterson or retrobulbar block. The auriculopalpebral nerve can be palpated as it crosses the zygomatic arch, roughly 5 cm to 6 cm behind the supraorbital process. Inject 5 mL of 2% lidocaine HCl subcutaneously on the dorsal aspect of the zygomatic arch at this location.

Peterson Nerve Block

After performing a small local skin block over the intended site of puncture, a 3.8-cm long, 14-gauge needle is inserted through the skin as a cannula for introduction of an 18-gauge, 9-cm long needle for the nerve block. The cannula is inserted caudal to the junction of the supraorbital process and zygomatic arch and is introduced through the skin. Then, the 18-gauge, 9-cm long needle is introduced through the cannula needle and is directed in a horizontal and slightly dorsal direction until the coronoid process is encountered. The needle is "walked off" the rostral aspect of the coronoid process and advanced in a ventromedial direction along the caudal aspect of the orbit until the needle encounters the bony plate encasing the foramen orbitorotundum. Once the needle is advanced to the foramen, it is advised that the needle be drawn back a few millimeters to reduce the risk of intrameningeal injection. After aspirating to assure the needle is not in the internal maxillary artery, 10 mL to 15 mL of lidocaine (2%) is deposited, with an additional 5 mL of lidocaine deposited as the needle is slowly withdrawn. Mydriasis indicates a successful block.

4-Point Retrobulbar Nerve Block

The 4-point retrobulbar block is technically easier and can be done more rapidly as compared with the Peterson eye block. In this technique, an 18-gauge, 9-cm long needle is introduced through the skin on the dorsal, lateral, ventral and medial aspects of the eye, at 12-, 3-, 6-, and 9-o'clock positions, respectively. Introduction of the needle through the conjunctiva should be avoided to reduce the occurrence of ocular contamination. The needle is directed behind the globe using the bony orbit as a guide. When the needle is introduced into retrobulbar sheath, the eye will move slightly with the tug of the needle. After this location is reached and aspiration is performed to assure that the needle is not in a vessel, 5 mL to 10 mL of lidocaine (2%) is deposited at each site. Mydriasis indicates a successful block.

Retrobulbar Block

An alternative to the 4-point retrobulbar block is the single retrobulbar block (**Fig. 2**). In this technique, the 9-cm long 18-gauge needle is bent into a half circle. The needle is inserted immediately ventral to the dorsal orbital rim and directed such that the needle impacts into the bone of the orbit. Then the needle is advanced as it is rotated ventrally in a progressive manner, such that the needle remains in close proximity to the bone. After the needle is inserted to the caudal aspect of the eye, 20 mL of 2% lidocaine HCl is administered after aspiration to ensure that the needle is not positioned in a vessel or other fluid structure. Successful deposition of lidocaine causes mild proptosis of the globe.

Ring Block

Additional local anesthesia of the eyelids is recommended as the Peterson and retrobulbar blocks typically result in incomplete analgesia of the eyelids. Five to 10 mL lidocaine (2%) is infiltrated subcutaneously 2.5 cm from the eyelid margins as a ring block.

Lidocaine Toxicity

Particular care should be taken in young calves not to exceed the toxic dose of lidocaine (10 mg/kg). This calculates out to 50 mL of 2% lidocaine per 100 kg of body weight (50 mL per 220 lbs body weight). Dilution of 2% lidocaine in saline can facilitate ease of distribution when restricted amounts are necessary.

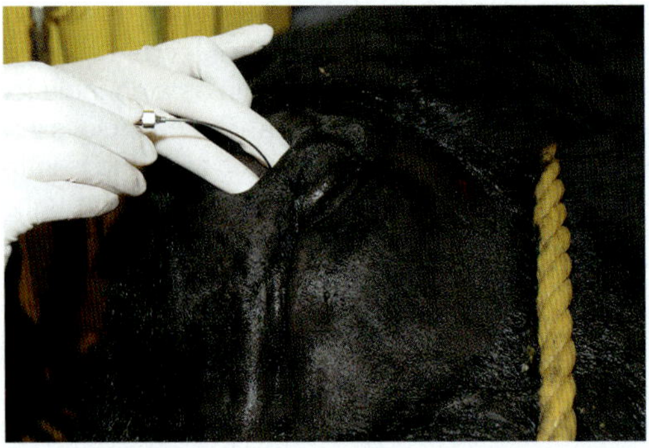

Fig. 2. Local anesthesia applied using a 3.5-inch 18-gauge needle bent into a half-circle for injection of lidocaine extensively in the retrobulbar space. (*Courtesy of* David Adams, Manhattan, KS and David E. Anderson, DVM, MS, Manhattan, KS.)

PERIOPERATIVE MANAGEMENT

Anti-Inflammatory and Analgesic Therapy

The disease process and degree of invasiveness will determine the degree of anti-inflammatory therapy required. Flunixin meglumine (1 mg/kg IV) immediately before surgical excision usually is adequate for enucleation procedures; however, further anti-inflammatory management may be warranted depending on the disease process and extent of excision.

Antibiotic Therapy

Because of the typical field conditions present during enucleation procedures, broad spectrum systemic antibiotic therapy is indicated. The disease process will dictate the duration of antibiotic therapy. Although there have been no publications regarding the placement of intraorbital suspensions or boluses, clinical observation of abscess with drainage after this practice cautions against the use of any material that may act as a future nidus of infection or that may cause inflammation or exacerbation of pain because of caustic or chemical effects. Systemic antibiotics combined with general surgical asepsis are likely to be the most efficacious therapeutic option.

SURGICAL TECHNIQUE

Suture

Absorbable sutures (eg, polyglecaprone No. 0) should be used for any ligation or subcutaneous procedure. Skin should be closed with an appropriately sized nonabsorbable suture (eg, nylon No. 3 or polymerized caprolactam No. 6) placed in a Ford-interlocking suture pattern or tension relieving suture patterns (eg, cruciate pattern).

Enucleation

A transpalpebral ablation technique is used to remove the eye. The upper and lower eyelids are sutured closed or alternatively, eyelids can be closed using multiple towel clamps (**Fig. 3**). A circumferential skin incision is made approximately 1 cm from the edges of the eyelids (**Fig. 4**). Using a combination of blunt and sharp dissection, Mayo scissors are used to dissect through the orbicularis oculi muscle, fascia, and subcutaneous tissue surrounding the eye. The interior of the bony orbit is used as a guide. The medial and lateral canthal ligaments are sharply transected to allow access to the caudal aspect of the orbit. As there is a large vessel associated with

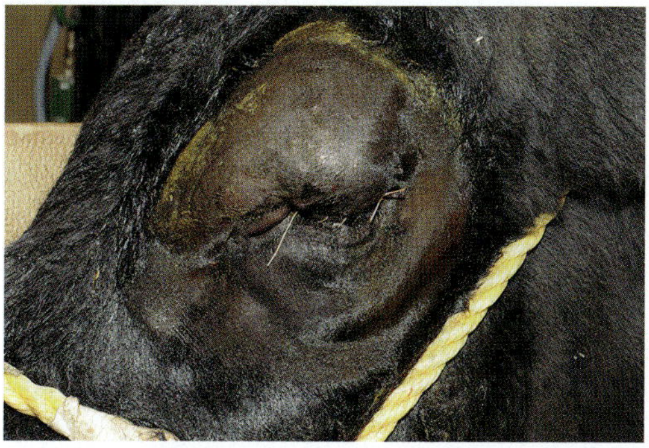

Fig. 3. Eyelids sutured closed using No. 2 PG-910 in a Ford interlocking pattern. (*Courtesy of* David Adams, Manhattan, KS and David E. Anderson, DVM, MS, Manhattan, KS.)

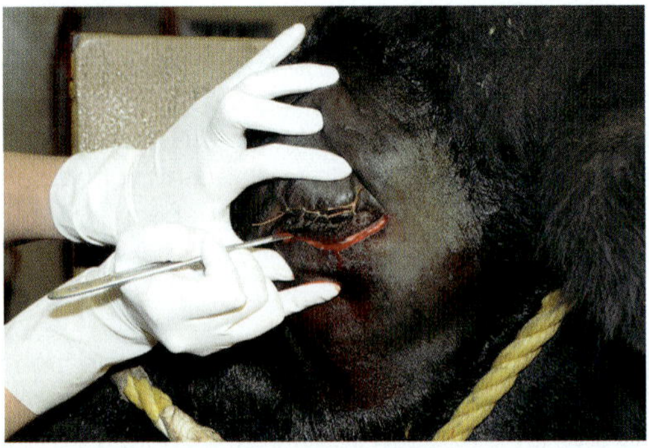

Fig. 4. Elliptic incision is made approximately 1-cm distant to eyelid suture margin. (*Courtesy of* David Adams, Manhattan, KS and David E. Anderson, DVM, MS, Manhattan, KS.)

the medial canthus, transection of the medial canthal ligaments is best left until necessary. Complete excision of orbital tissue is necessary in most cases of eye removal. The retrobulbar musculature and the optic nerve sheath should be transected as far caudally as feasible (**Fig. 5**). A vascular clamp can aid in hemostasis while additional excision of remaining orbital tissue is undertaken. In cases where neoplastic infiltration of the bony orbit has occurred, affected areas of ocular periosteum should be thoroughly excised. An orbitotomy may be necessary to remove affected areas of orbital bone; however radical resection of orbital bone and associated lymph nodes is an extensive procedure not recommended except in tertiary care setting.[8]

The skin incision can be closed in a variety of patterns with a nonabsorbable suture, such as No. 3 nylon. Common patterns include the Ford interlocking, cruciate, or simple continuous (**Fig. 6**). An interrupted suture should be placed in the medial canthal portion of the skin closure to allow for facilitation of drainage if necessary.

If a cosmetic result is desired, a "trampoline" suture can be employed to reduce the hollow appearance of the orbit. However, it is not recommended in cases where there is periorbital infection or neoplasia present. Placement of a trampoline suture is done by grasping the periosteum on the dorsal and ventral rim of the orbit using a simple continuous pattern with No. 2 polypropylene or equivalent nonabsorbable suture.

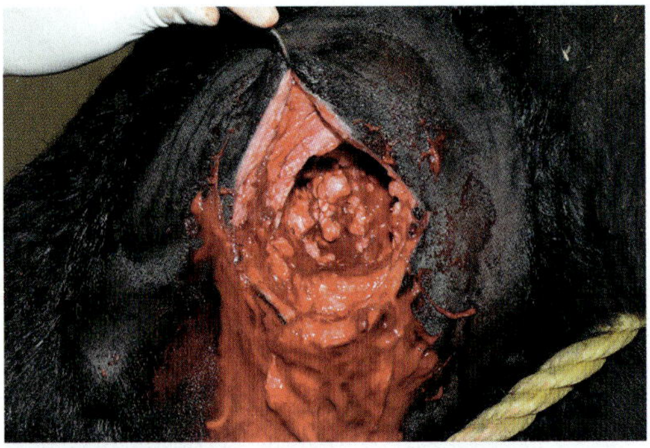

Fig. 5. Empty orbit after excision of globe. Optic pedicle has been ligated using No. 2-0 PG-910. (*Courtesy of* David Adams, Manhattan, KS and David E. Anderson, DVM, MS, Manhattan, KS.)

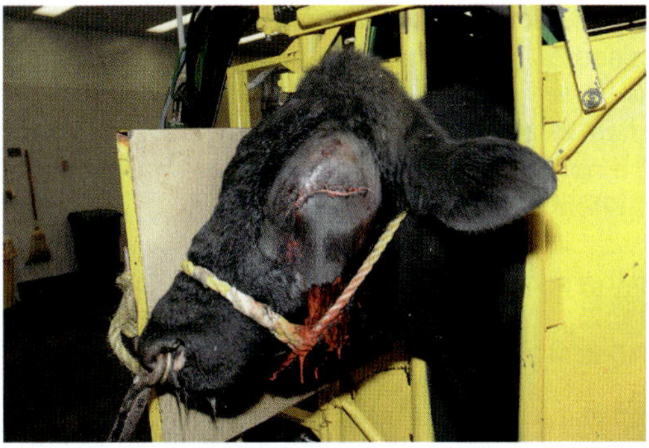

Fig. 6. Skin sutured closed using No. 6 Nylon in Ford interlocking pattern. (*Courtesy of* David Adams, Manhattan, KS and David E. Anderson, DVM, MS, Manhattan, KS.)

The sutures are tightened to allow for support of the overlying ocular skin. The skin is subsequently sutured using a Ford interlocking, cruciate, or simple continuous pattern and No. 2 or No. 3 nylon suture. The skin sutures are removed routinely in 14 to 21 days, leaving the underlying trampoline sutures in place as a permanent support.

POSTOPERATIVE CARE

The animal should be kept in a confined area for several days after surgery to allow for appropriate hemostasis to occur. Daily observation of the surgical site and assessment of general well being is recommended until suture removal. Sutures should be removed in 14 to 21 days to allow for complete healing of the skin.

Postoperative Complications

Postoperative complications can include simple incisional infection, orbital infections, dehiscence of the suture, significant infections of the periorbital tissue, or progression of neoplasia into bone or regional lymph nodes. Cattle often demonstrate pruritis after surgery, which can lead to incisional dehiscence because of head rubbing. If purulent drainage is noted during the course of healing in an enucleation procedure, the medial interrupted suture may be removed and the cavity flushed with a dilute disinfectant solution daily until resolution of the orbital infection. Antibiotic therapy is recommended if systemic signs of infection are noted.

H-BLEPHAROPLASTY

For invasive eyelid lesions where greater than one-third of the lower eyelid is involved, straightforward surgical excision of the mass is not advised. A sliding skin graft procedure, the H-blepharoplasty can be performed in these cases to remove the affected tissue and create a functional lower eyelid margin.[9] The procedure is relatively easy to perform in selected candidates.

Two full thickness skin incisions are made perpendicular to the eyelid margin on either side of the mass, extending beyond the mass approximately the length of the mass. A full thickness skin incision parallel to the eyelid margin is made at the base of the eyelid mass, connecting the two initial vertical skin incisions, thus creating an H shape. Two equilateral triangular pieces of skin exterior to the intended graft are then removed, extending from the horizontal crossbar to the base of the vertical incisions of the graft to allow for movement of the graft toward the eyelid margin. The mass is excised from the underlying subcutaneous tissue via dissection using Mayos or Metzembaum scissors. To create the sliding graft, the base of the H is then dissected free from the underlying subcutaneous tissue. The graft is placed in alignment with the original vertical skin incisions and the eyelid margin. The graft is sutured to the skin incisions using a nonabsorbable suture in an interrupted pattern. The eyelid margin is typically left to heal by second intention.

Sutures are removed in 14 to 21 days and care is taken to assure the animal does not excessively rub the surgical site during the healing period.

RETROBULBAR FAT PAD REMOVAL

Prolapse of the retrobulbar fat pad is an uncommon but relatively striking disorder diagnosed by visual appraisal and digital examination. If surgical intervention is required, either because of aesthetics or visual compromise, the fad pad is easily removed with the aid of an auriculopalpabral nerve block and topical anesthetic. After appropriate restraint and anesthesia, a small incision is made through the conjunctiva enveloping the retrobulbar fat. The fat is excised using a Mayo scissors. If possible, the ensuing rent in the conjunctiva can be closed using small absorbable suture in a simple interrupted or continuous pattern (eg, polyglycolic acid No. 3-0).

REFERENCES

1. Bistner S, Gastavo A, Batik G. Diseases of the orbit. In: Bistner S, Gastavo A, Batik G, editors. Atlas of veterinary ophthalmic surgery. Philadelphia: WB Saunders; 1977. p. 265–77.
2. Brooks DE. Orbit. In: Auer J, Stick J, editors. Equine surgery. 2nd edition. Philadelphia: Saunders; 1999. p. 497–514.
3. Irby NL. Surgical diseases of the eye in farm animals. In: Fubini S, Ducharme NG, editors. Farm animal surgery. St. Louis (MO): Saunders; 2004. p. 429–59.
4. Ivany JM. Farm animal anesthesia. In: Fubini S, Ducharme NG, editors. Farm animal surgery. St. Louis (MO): Saunders; 2004. p. 97–112.
5. Slatter D. Orbit. In: Kersey R, editor. Fundamentals of veterinary ophthalmology. 3rd edition. Philadelphia: WB Saunders; 2001. p. 516–31.
6. Muir MW. Local anesthesia in ruminants and pigs. In: Schrefer J, editor. Handbook of veterinary anesthesia. 4th edition. St. Louis (MO): Mosby; 2005. p. 72–99.
7. Rubin LF. Large animal ophthalmic surgery. In: Jennings P Jr, editor. The practice of large animal surgery, Vol. II. Philadelphia: Saunders; 1984. p. 1151–201.
8. Klein WR, Bier J, van Dieten JS, et al. Radical surgery of bovine ocular squamous cell carcinoma (cancer eye): complications and results. Vet Surg 1984;13:236–42.
9. Welker B, Modransky PD, Hoffsis GF, et al. Excision of neoplasms of the bovine lower eyelid by H-blepharoplasty. Vet Surg 1991;20(2):133–9.

Surgical Diseases and Techniques of the Digit

André Desrochers, DMV, MS[a,*], David E. Anderson, DVM, MS[b], Guy St. Jean, DMV, MS[c]

KEYWORDS

- Surgery • Cattle • Digit • Lameness • Resection
- Amputation • Septic arthritis

Claw diseases in cattle are common under field conditions. Sole ulcer, sole abscess, foot-rot, digital dermatitis, and interdigital dermatitis are frequently diagnosed and treated by owners, foot trimmers, and veterinarians. Surgical digital diseases include vertical cracks, septic arthritis of the distal and proximal interphalangeal joints, tenosynovitis and flexor tendon necrosis, pedal osteomyelitis, interdigital hyperplesia, phalangeal luxation, distal phalanx fracture, and degenerative joint diseases of the coffin joint. Most digital surgical conditions are manageable in field conditions. However, some postoperative care is more demanding and, therefore, prevents some veterinarians from performing such techniques in field conditions. Even if most techniques are easy to perform, nevertheless surgical decision making, perioperative treatment, and pain management are more challenging than the technique itself. Knowledge and understanding of the digital anatomy is essential before performing surgeries. Readers are referred to anatomy textbooks and other book chapters for more information on this topic.[1–3]

RESTRAIN, ANESTHESIA, AND PREPARATION

Most of the following procedures can be performed with the animal standing in a trimming chute. However, if the dorsal aspect of the foot has to be dissected, then this procedure would be easier to perform with the animal in lateral recumbency. Diseases and surgical interventions of the foot are painful. Adequate analgesia and anesthesia

[a] Department of Clinical Sciences, Université de Montréal, C.P. 5000 Saint-Hyacinthe, Quebec J2S 7C6, Canada
[b] Department of Clinical Sciences, College of Veterinary Medicine, Kansas State University, 1800 Dennison Avenue, Manhattan, KS 66506, USA
[c] School of Veterinary Medicine, Ross University, P.O. Box 334, Basseterre, Saint-Kitts, West Indies
* Corresponding author.
E-mail address: andre.desrochers@umontreal.ca (A. Desrochers).

Vet Clin Food Anim 24 (2008) 535–550
doi:10.1016/j.cvfa.2008.07.005 **vetfood.theclinics.com**
0749-0720/08/$ – see front matter © 2008 Elsevier Inc. All rights reserved.

are essential for patient comfort and surgeon comfort, as well as for improving surgical manipulations. Anesthetic procedures frequently used for foot surgery are intravenous lidocaine under tourniquet and the 4-point digital block.

Surgical instruments needed for digit surgery are basic. Specific instruments to debride infected joints or to perform joint amputation will be pointed out for the different procedures discussed. However, it is important to mention that orthopedic-grade surgical instruments are not necessary in field conditions.

If necessary, a block can be glued to the sound claw with polymethylmethacrylate (PMMA) before extensive debridement and the surgical preparation. Surgical preparation should be performed as with any other surgery, being sure to clean the interdigital cleft. The nonaffected digit can be covered with a latex glove if the dirt is difficult to remove, or if it is necessary to cover a wooden block. While the animal is standing in a trimming chute, a large plastic bag can be attached on each side of the back of the chute to avoid urination and defecation on the surgical site.

DISTAL INTERPHALANGEAL JOINT INFECTION

Sepsis of the distal interphalageal (DIP) joint is caused mainly by extension of sole diseases, such as sole abscesses and white-line disease. A penetrating foreign body in the interdigital space or foot-rot is also often implicated in sepsis of the DIP joint. In dairy cattle, the origin of DIP sepsis is most likely sole ulcers, while in beef cattle the cause is often unknown. The distal sesamoid bone and its bursa, the tendinous portion of the deep digital flexor (DDF) muscle, the tendon sheath of the DDF muscle, and the superficial digital flexor muscles are in close relationship and solar infection can rapidly spread to these structures. The history of affected cattle is often typical: they have history of chronic lameness being treated unsuccessfully for foot-rot or sole ulcer. Severity of the lameness is quite variable, depending of the extent of infection and the chronicity of the disease.

The hallmarks of DIP infection are a swollen and painful coronary band with a draining tract, either at the proximal aspect of the coronary band or under the sole (**Fig. 1**). A swollen heel suggests infection of the distal sesamoid bone and its bursa and the digital cushion pad, and a fistula tract may be present at the heel skin junction (**Fig. 2**). Cattle with deep sepsis of the digit show sign of pain when the heel is palpated or the digit is extended. The tendinous portion of the DDF tendon might rupture if the necrotic process is severe, and the digit affected will tilt upward (**Fig. 3**).

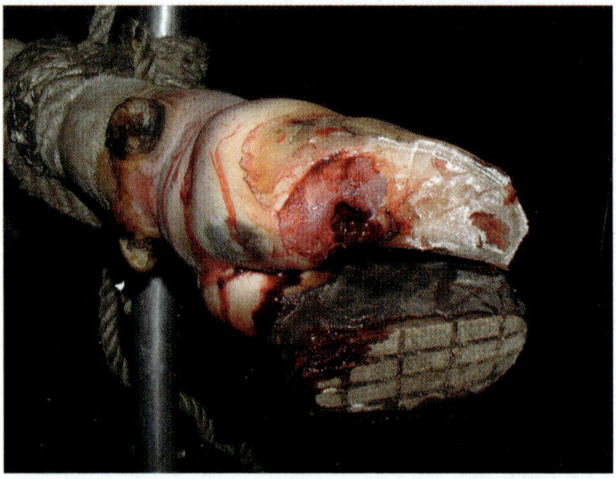

Fig. 1. Holstein adult cow suffering of a chronic infected sole ulcer. The coronary band and the heel are swollen.

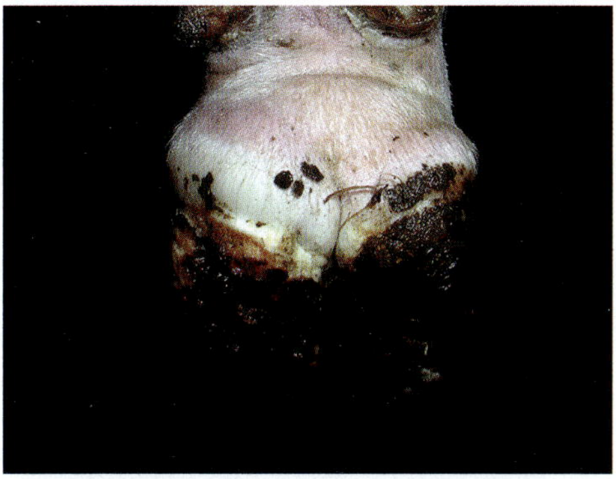

Fig. 2. Holstein adult cow with a swollen heel and an enlarged pastern.

Radiographic evaluation of the DIP joint is helpful to determine the extent and duration of the process. Usually the lesions are not subtle because of the chronicity of the infection. Radiographic views of a DIP joint with chronic septic arthritis show an increased joint space because of subchondral bone lysis (**Fig. 4**). Distal and proximal periosteal proliferation is present. The distal sesamoid bone may show lysis of its articular surface or may be destroyed completely. The proximal interphalangeal (PIP) joint might also be involved in the process. If a fistula tract is present, communication with the DIP joint is confirmed with the insertion of a sterile probe into the tract. Recently, ultrasonography was investigated as a diagnostic method for DIP joint sepsis. When compared with the partner sound claw, the dorsal pouch of the infected DIP joint was larger. With a linear probe applied longitudinally on the dorsal aspect of the digit, it was determined that the infected joint had a dorsal pouch greater than 6 mm.[4]

Acute septic arthritis of the DIP joint is rare but possible. Athrocentesis is indicated, and synovial fluid may be submitted for cytologic examination and bacterial culture. Treatment consists of systemic and local antibiotics and thorough joint lavage with

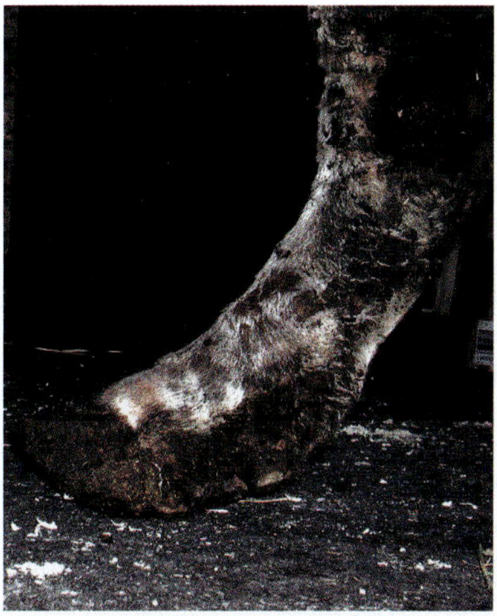

Fig. 3. Adult Charolais bull presented for chronic lameness of the left hind limb. The lateral digit of the left foot is tilted upward, indicating a rupture of the deep flexor tendon. The bull was diagnosed with sepsis of the DIP joint.

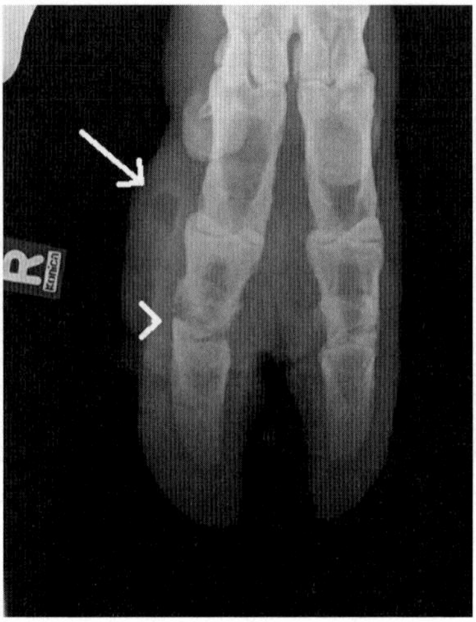

Fig. 4. Radiographic image of a distal right foot. This dorsoplantar view shows swelling of the lateral digit (*white arrow*) and subchondral bone lysis of the distal interphalangeal joint.

14-gauge, 5-cm needles inserted dorsoproximal to the coronary band, axial or abaxial to the tendinous portion of the extensor muscle, and with an angle of 60° to the coronary band. Lavage of the joint is performed until the synovial fluid is clear and without fibrin clots. Arthrotomy should be considered if fibrin is abundant and lavage difficult.

Chronic presentation of septic arthritis of the DIP joint is a more common situation. Conservative treatment with systemic antibiotics and a wooden block on the sound claw is often ineffective. Surgery is the treatment of choice to provide debridement and drainage of the DIP joint. The two surgical options are digit amputation and joint resection.

DIGIT AMPUTATION

Digit amputation has been used successfully to treat pedal osteitis, luxation or fracture of the distal phalanx, deep sepsis of the digit, and septic arthritis of the DIP or PIP joint. The advantages are that it is a rapid and inexpensive procedure, all the infected tissues are resected, and cattle usually return rapidly to their previous level of production.[5–7] The disadvantages are that the expected production life might be reduced, heavy animals are reported to do poorly, and the cosmetic result is poor. The production life of cattle that have a digit amputated depends on which digit was removed, the weight of the animal, and the type of housing. Production longevity of cattle after digit amputation ranges between 10 and 27 months.[6,8,9] Cattle weighing more than 680 kg that have a digit amputated will have a short production life.[6] Recently, Starke showed that no significant difference was found in survival time between digit amputation (27.2 months) and joint resection (21.2 months) in bulls.[9] However, the survival time in dairy cattle affected by DIP joint sepsis and treated by amputation was 13.5 months, compared with 10.9 months for the joint resection group, but the results were not statistically significant.[10] Bicalho and colleagues compared amputation and arthrodesis of the DIP joint in a control study on lactating cows.[11] The failure rate—defined as culled in less than 60 days of milking after the surgery—was 44.9%, compared with 0% for the arthrodesis group. Yield milk production was higher for cattle that underwent arthrodesis, compared with the amputation group. They concluded that arthrodesis should be favored.

The site of amputation should be chosen based on the extent of the infection. Digit amputation through the distal aspect of the proximal phalanx is the most common technique. It is a rapid and simple procedure and usually provides a wide resection and effective drainage of the affected digit and the flexor tendon sheath. The wound is further away from the ground, compared with a low amputation preventing ulceration. However, a low amputation will provide more digital stability because the interdigital cruciate ligament is preserved. Desarticulation or amputation through the joint is an easy technique to do in field situation.[11] If the cartilage of the phalanx is left intact after disarticulation, coverage by granulation tissue might be delayed and cyst-like lesions might form as well.[12]

The distal limb is prepared surgically and intravenous regional anesthesia is administered. The interdigital skin is incised to the level of the PIP joint or the very distal aspect of the proximal phalanx axially. A gigli wire is inserted in the interdigital space with an angle of 45° to the proximal digit abaxially (**Fig. 5**). An assistant can hold the digit to provide more stability when the cut is performed. The cut should go through the distal portion of the proximal phalanx. The interdigital fat and all remaining necrotic tissues are removed. Digital vessels are ligatured with absorbable suture as needed. The wound is lavaged and dried. A semiocclusive layer is applied on the distal portion of the proximal phalanx, multiple layers of gauze are put over it and it is then wrapped with adhesive bandage. The bandage is changed 24 hours after the surgery and then changed again every 4 to 5 days, as needed. Ideally, bandages are continued until the surface of the bone is covered with granulation tissue. A broad spectrum, systemic antibiotic is administered for 5 to 10 days after the surgery. It should be remembered that antibiotics will never replace good surgical principals and adequate postoperative hygiene. Bulls can return to breeding 3 to 4 months after the surgery.

A skin flap could be preserved to cover the stump by continuing the interdigital incision distal and abaxial at the palmar and dorsal aspect of the digit and along the proximal aspect of the coronary band.[12] Although this technique provides a superior

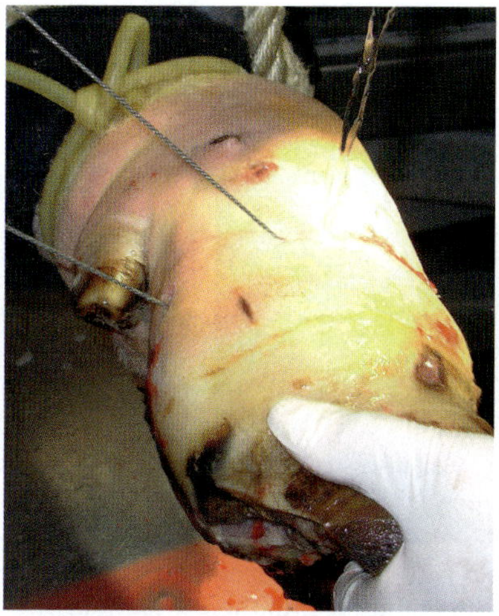

Fig. 5. An amputation through the proximal phalanx is performed with the animal on lateral recumbency. The gigli wire is at 45° and crossed to allow a better cut.

cosmetic result and decreases subsequent care of the stump, it may prevent adequate drainage and extension of the infection. This technique is recommended for a nonseptic process of the digit (pedal fracture, digit luxation) or distal sepsis without extensive soft tissue infection (pedal osteitis). If a skin flap is elected in the presence of infection, the distal portion of the incision should be left opened for drainage (**Fig. 6**).

RESECTION OF THE DIP JOINT

The techniques for resection of the DIP joint differ by surgical approach. Choice of a technique should be based on the anatomic structure infected and the location of existing draining tracts. Intact ligaments and tendons should be preserved, when possible, to keep the affected digit stable during the ankylosis process. However, if necrotic tendinitis and tendon sheath septis are present, then extensive surgical exposure might be necessary to debride and control the infection of the foot. Inadequate examination and diagnosis will either delay healing or the animal will not respond to treatment. The advantages and disadvantages of resection of the DIP joint compared with digit amputation are that cattle have discussed in the digit amputation.

Resection of the DIP Joint: Solar Approach

The purpose of the resection is to provide drainage, debriding the necroting tissue, and removing the articular cartilage favoring ankylosis. The surgery is performed under sedation and intravenous regional anesthesia or regional nerve block. Cattle are restrained in a foot-trimming chute or in lateral recumbency with the affected leg uppermost. The plantar or palmar portion of the sole and the heel should be pared away until the sole can be indented easily. In severe and extensive infection of the DIP joint originating from a solar lesion, the distal sesamoid bone and the joint can be felt through the wound and the sole already can be indented easily. The distal limb is

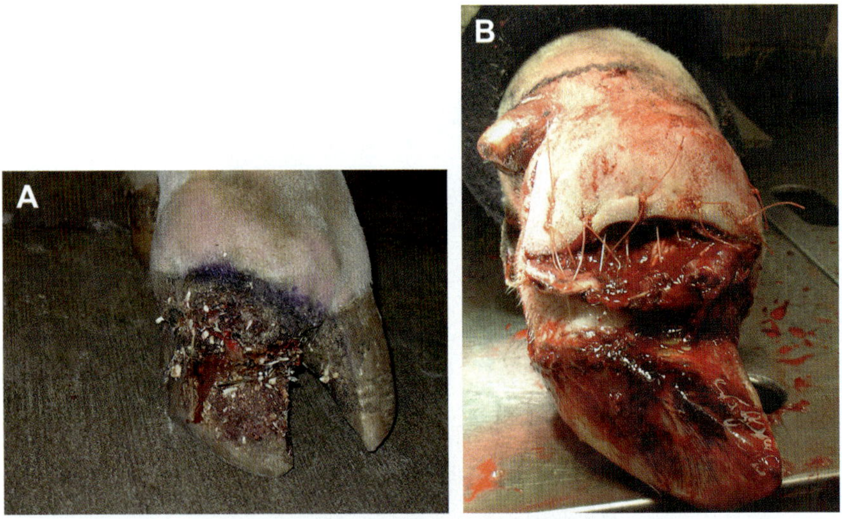

Fig. 6. (*A*) Animal presented with a severe chronic laceration of the lateral digit. The laceration was infected and communicating with the DIP joint. (*B*) The digit was amputated and a flap of skin re-covered the proximal digit but the distal portion of the incision was left open for drainage.

prepared surgically. An elliptic incision is made around the necrotic area at the sole and heel junction. The width of the incision should be close to the axial and abaxial white line. The proximal portion of the elliptic incision is joined just before crossing the coronary band, avoiding cutting a wedge of it. Depending of the extent of infection, the elliptic incision is extended proximally as far as needed. The incision can be extended proximal to the accessory digit by making the incision on the axial side of the accessory digits.[3,12,13] The tendinous portion of DDF muscle is cut from its insertion on the distal phalanx and resected proximally up to 2 cm to 3 cm or more if necrotic. The distal sesamoid bone is then exposed. If the sesamoid bone is necrotic, it can be easily removed with a rongeur. If not, the two collateral ligaments and the distal ligaments are resected with a scalpel blade. The DIP joint should be exposed at this point (**Fig. 7**). All necrotic tissue should be removed to speed up healing. Debridement of the joint from the solar wound can be performed with a curette, a hoof knife, or with a 5-mm to 13-mm drill bit. The drill exits through the dorsal wall, 1-cm distal to the coronary band (**Fig. 8**). Some authors prefer to exit proximal to the coronary band.[14] Wherever the drill bit exits, the coronary band must be avoided to prevent compromising future horn production. Even after the joint is drilled, necrotic tissue might still be present, so it has to be curetted thoroughly. Copious lavage is performed with isotonic solution. If the tendon sheath or the tendinous portion of the superficial digital flexor muscle is infected and necrotic, the incision can be extended 2 cm to 3 cm proximally to the accessory digit, allowing debridement and drainage (**Fig. 9**).

A wooden block is glued with PMMA on the healthy digit of the affected limb. The wound is bandaged and lavage is performed every other day, if possible. It is the authors' opinion that the infected digit should not be wired to the parent digit for immobilization purposes. By attaching the digits, the infected digit will be constantly moving, increasing the pain because of the movement and delaying the ankylosis process. Systemic antibiotics are given for 10 to 14 days, depending on adjacent soft tissue infection. Nonsteroidal anti-inflammatory drugs are given as needed for the first few days postoperatively.

Kostlin and Nuss[15] has reported a success rate of 85% for 281 cattle with this technique. This technique provides good visualization of the DIP joint, excellent drainage, and a good long-term prognosis. Variations of the solar approach are described in the literature. Some techniques are more invasive, with deep dissection of the plantar or

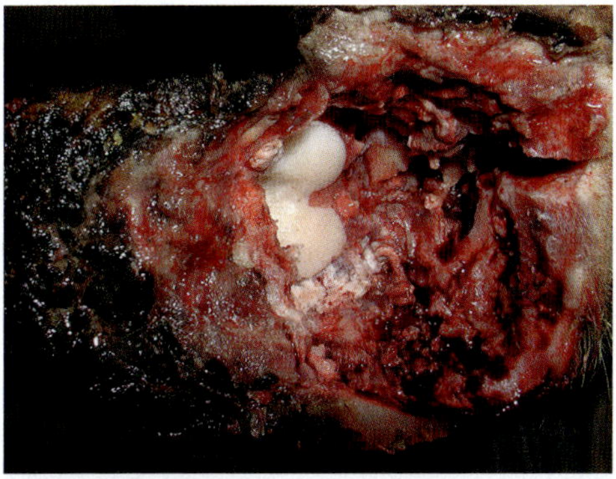

Fig. 7. Solar view of a digit undergoing DIP joint resection. The distal sesamoid bone was resected exposing the DIP joint. The plantar aspect of the distal condyles of the middle phalanx are seen through the wound.

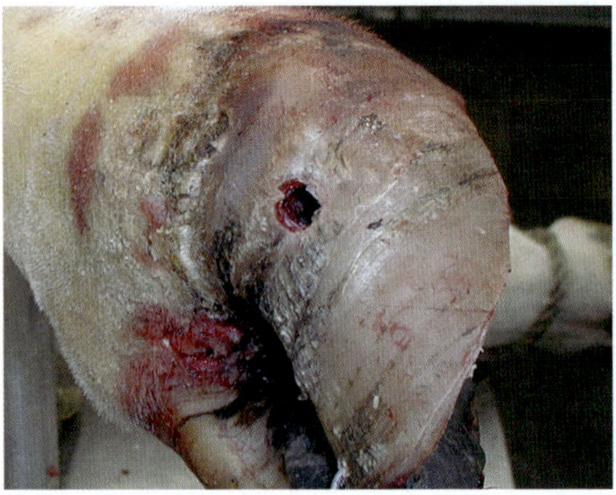

Fig. 8. Resection was performed by solar approach. A hole from the exit site of the drill bit is seen on the dorsal wall just distal to the coronary band.

palmar aspect of the digit, while other techniques consist only of providing drainage of the joint by drilling a hole through the joint. The extent of the infection should determine the technique to be used.

Resection of the DIP Joint: Bulbar Approach

This variation has been reported by Greenough.[5] The bulbar approach consists of a horizontal incision around the circumference of the heel 1-cm distal to the skin horn junction. A wedge of hypodermic tissue and tendon is resected, providing visualization of the distal sesamoid bone. The sesamoid bone is resected, as described before, and the digit is extended to provide a good visualization of the DIP joint (**Fig. 10**). After debridement and lavage of the joint, the incision can be sutured and bandaged. A wooden block is applied with PMMA on the healthy digit of the affected limb. This technique provides better visualization of the DIP joint without invading the tendon sheath when it is not necessary. Recently, Bicalho and colleagues described a modification of the technique where the incision is proximal to the coronary band.[16] If the deep digital flexor tendon is necrotic and the tendon sheath infected, then a second incision is made over the tendon through the tendon sheath, proximally to the accessory digits. First, the distal portion of the deep digital flexor tendon is pushed

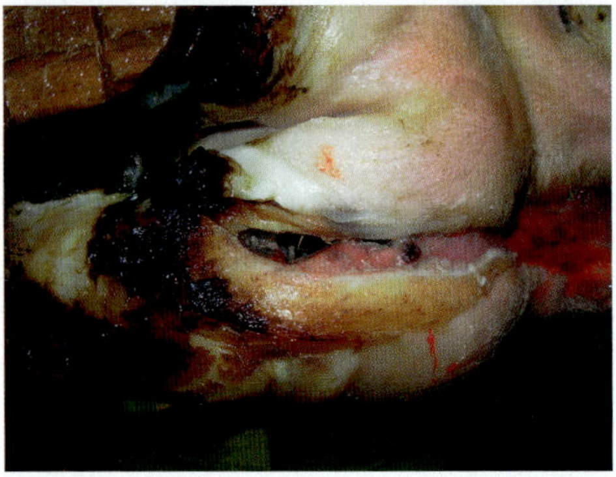

Fig. 9. Plantar view of a foot that underwent DIP joint resection and extensive tendon resection. This picture was taken 3 weeks postoperatively.

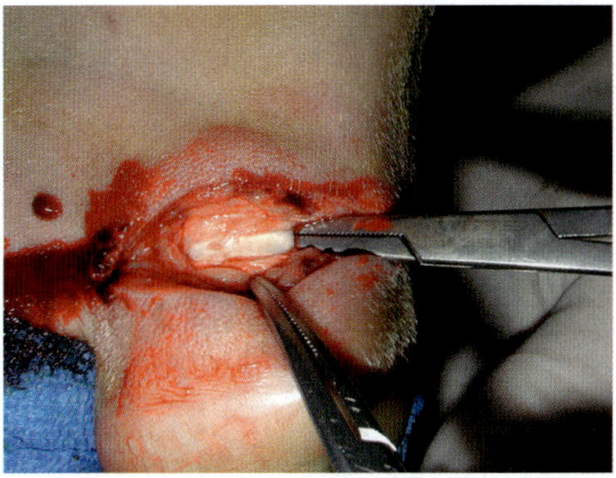

Fig. 10. Palmar approach of the DIP joint. Resection was performed to treat degenerative joint disease of the DIP joint on a 6-month-old Holstein heifer. In that particular case, the incision was made proximal to the coronary band. The tendon of the deep digital flexor tendon is about to be cut to get access to the DIP joint.

proximally in to the tendon sheath, then it is grabbed and pulled by the proximal incision. After joint resection, a drain could be passed through the incisions and attached on the abaxial aspect of the digit and the proximal incision is sutured (**Fig. 11**). Affected cattle were very lame for 2 weeks, but were sound within five months.[16]

The authors have been using the bulbar approach for resection of the DIP joint in nonseptic processes (degenerative joint disease of the DIP joint and laceration), avoiding disruption of the intact solar surface and decreasing chance of infection.[14]

RESECTION OF THE DIP BY ABAXIAL APPROACH

In this technique, an orthopedic drill with a 6-mm to 12-mm drill bit is used to create a tunnel through the abaxial hoof wall at the level of the DIP joint. The drill is passed through the DIP joint and exited through the dorsoaxial interdigital space distal to the coronary band.[17] The entry site for the drill bit is estimated as the intersection of two imaginary lines, one drawn parallel to the coronary band approximately one-third the distance from the coronary band to the sole and the other line drawn perpendicular

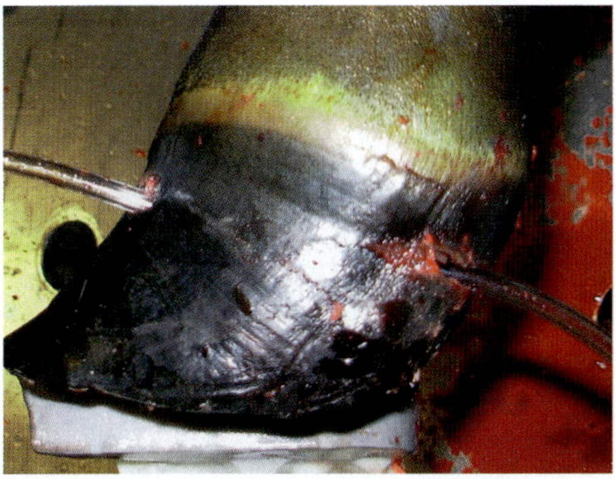

Fig. 11. A fenestrated plastic tubing was inserted through the entry holes made by the drill bit.

to the coronary band, approximately half of the distance from the heel bulb to the dorsal hoof wall. This approach is easy to perform, but the exit site of the drill bit is difficult to control, especially if the animal is not well restrained. Debridement of the cartilage and necrotic bone also is difficult to assess. The defect in the hoof wall remains open to facilitate drainage, thus the hoof wall is weakened by this technique. The authors have not observed specific hoof wall complications of this technique, but cattle should be confined to a small area with excellent footing during the early stages of healing.

Recently, Zulauf and colleagues[18] proposed an alternative to this method. They performed a precise abaxial hoof wall excision using a fine rotating burr. A hoof wall segment measuring approximately 15 mm by 40 mm was removed and the proximal margin of the defect was approximately 1-cm distal to the coronary band. This technique provides a relatively large, rectangular hoof wall defect through which to access the DIP joint. Although access to the joint is superior to the previously described technique, the defect size is substantial.

PROXIMAL INTERPHALANGEAL JOINT INFECTION

Septic arthritis of the PIP joint is secondary to a direct trauma, adjacent infection, or systemic infection in young animals (**Fig. 12**).[19] Affected animals are very lame and a fistula tract with necrotic tissue is often observed at the abaxial aspect of the pastern joint away from the coronary band. Diagnosis is based on physical examination, probing the lesion, or radiographic imaging of the digit. This condition should be treated surgically with extensive debridement of the joint or amputation.

Choice of surgical technique is based on the extent of the infection. If infection is limited to the PIP joint, resection of the joint should be favored. However, if the flexor tendon sheath and DIP joint are also infected, then high amputation has to be considered. Abaxial existing wound or draining tract is used to access the joint. Arthrotomies should always be performed on the abaxial or dorsal aspect to avoid tendons and major blood vessels (**Fig. 13**). The joint is easily debrided with a curette until hard bone can be felt. The joint is lavaged as needed for a few days and the wound protected from environmental contamination until the athrotomy sites are filled with sound granulation tissues (**Fig. 14**). The prognosis is considered good.[19]

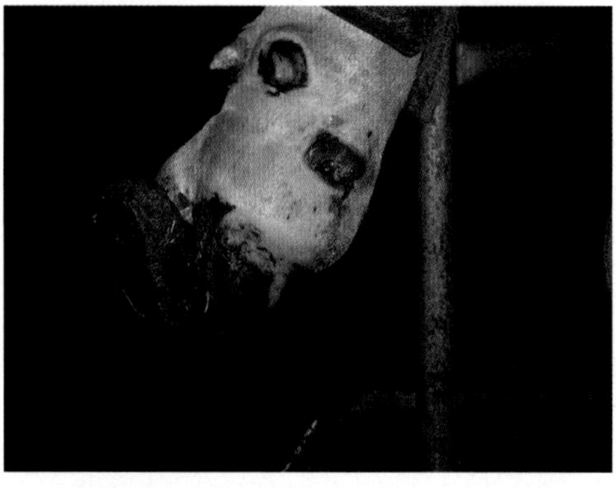

Fig. 12. PIP joint sepsis. A draining tract is observed on the abaxial aspect of the lateral digit at the pastern level. The digit is swollen.

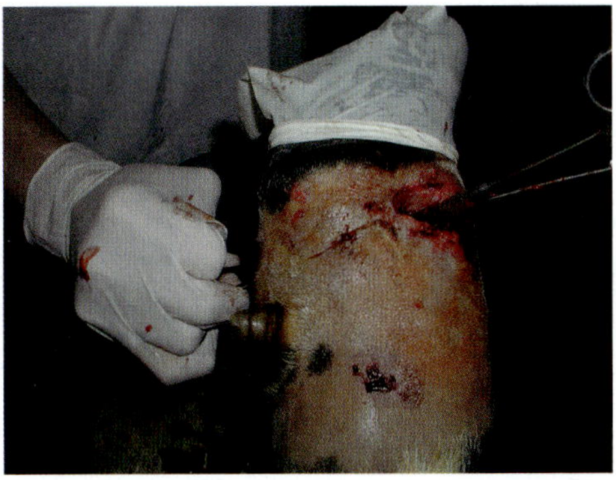

Fig. 13. This adult cow was suffering from PIP joint sepsis. Joint resection is performed with an abaxial approach.

PEDAL OSTEOMYELITIS

Pedal osteomyelitis is defined as a septic process of the distal phalanx. The infection originates from a solar trauma (such as puncture wound or severe abrasion at the toe) extension of an existing infection around the distal phalanx. The incidence could be high in feedlot cattle on a concrete floor. Cattle recently placed in a feedlot will fight around a feed bunk and their hind digits will slip on the concrete floor, causing severe abrasion at the toe region and secondary infection. Over-trimming with a grinding disc is also a cause of apical necrosis, as described by Kofler (**Fig. 15**).[20]

A preoperative radiograph is helpful to evaluate the extent of the infection. The DIP joint and the flexor tendon sheath should be examined. The surgical approach is based on the adjacent structure involved. The sole, infected corium and the distal phalanx are debrided with a curette and rongeur until sound hard bone is felt. A detached claw wall from the corion should not be left in place and subtotal resection is often necessary to provide better healing and improve walking (**Fig. 16**). Hoof nippers can

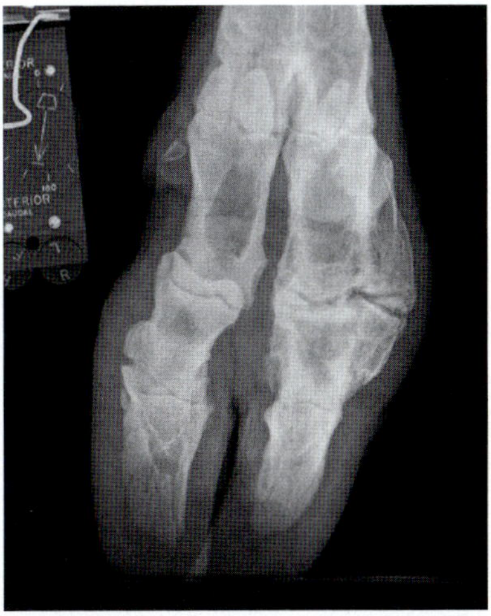

Fig. 14. Radiographic view of a foot (dorsoplantar view). The animal was treated surgically for a PIP sepsis 1 year ago. The PIP joint of the medial digit is ankylosed. Although a joint space can still be seen, the joint was immobile and the animal perfectly sound.

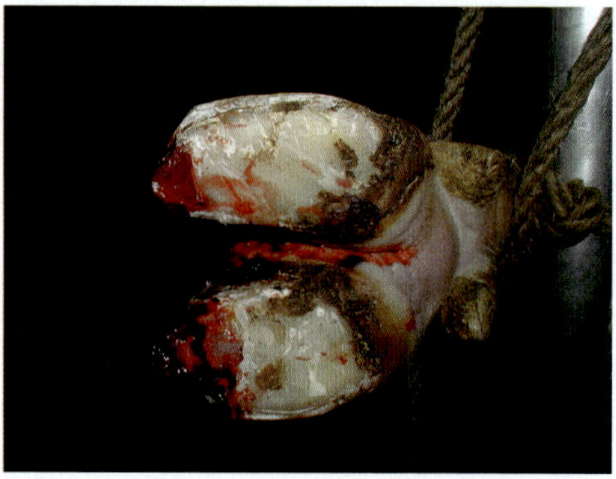

Fig. 15. Severe apical necrosis of both digit of a hind limb. Subtotal resection of the claws have to be performed to control the osteomyelitis of the distal phalanx.

be used to cut the affected apical portion of the claw.[3] Lavage is performed and the wound is bandaged. A wooden block is applied on the healthy digit of the affected limb. Bandaging and lavage should be continued until the infection is controlled and granulation tissue covers the distal phalanx.

The DIP joint can become infected by bacterial translocation. The infected joint can be either resected or amputated. The approach for joint resection might differ, depending of the location of the pedal lesion.

INTERDIGITAL HYPERPLASIA

Interdigital hyperplasia is a proliferative reaction of the interdigital skin. Excessive outward spreading of the digits, secondary to an underdeveloped ligamentous structure, overstretches the interdigital skin and causes hyperplasia.[21] Interdigital hyperplasia may be hereditary in Hereford and Fresian breeds. Males are more often affected than females.[22] Interdigital necrobacillosis and interdigital and digital dermatitis

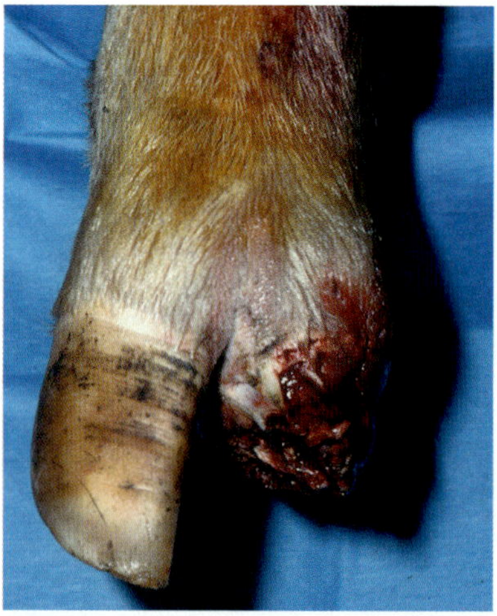

Fig. 16. This heifer was treated for severe pedal osteomyelitis. Two-thirds of the distal phalanx were resected. A wooden block was unnecessary because the affected digit was already elevated.

have been implicated in the etiology of interdigital hyperplasia.[23] Recently, Holzhauer and colleagues[24] reported the evolution of digital dermatitis lesions in an endemically affected dairy herd. Digital dermatitis lesions were present in all cows diagnosed with interdigtal hyperplasia.

Cattle affected with interdigital hyperplasia may be moderately to severely lame. The lesion is malodorous if associated with digital dermatitis or if secondary infection is present. The proliferative mass is hairless, ulcerated secondary to pressure trauma, and foreign materials may be present between the mass and the axial border of the digits. The protruding growth itself is not painful; however, the animal will react to successive flexion, abduction, and extension of the digits. The hyperplasia is typically present at the dorsal aspect of the interdigital space along the coronary band (**Fig. 17**). In some animals the lesion is off to the coronary band. In the authors' experience, these lesions are less troublesome than the axially centered overgrowth. Often adjacent, even emerging from the axial coronary band, their anatomic situation preclude resection because of possible invasion of the DIP joint. The hind limbs are affected most often, and the lesions can be found on one limb or all four limbs. Although heritability of this disease is controversial, young bulls affected with interdigital hyperplasia should be carefully examined to find the cause.

En bloc resection of the growth can be performed easily in a field situation. Surgery is better performed with the animal on lateral recumbency because of easier access to the dorsal aspect of the interdigital cleft where the mass is larger. Anesthesia is achieved either by 4-point digital block, intravenous lidocaine under tourniquet, or simply interdigital infiltration of lidocaine. If the interdigital injection is favored, the needle should be inserted proximal and dorsal to the mass. If en bloc resection is chosen, an Allis or LaHey tissue forcep is used to hold the corn (**Fig. 18**). A wedge-shaped excision is made on each side of the mass through the interdigital skin. All hyperplastic tissues should be removed because of possible recurrence. If full thickness is achieved, the interdigital fat will protrude from the incision. The interdigital fat should be removed to avoid its interposition between the skin edges and delay healing. Hemorrhage is controlled and a bandage is applied. The toes are wired together by drilling two holes through the hoof wall at the point of the toes to facilitate healing. The bandage is left in place for 5 days and the animal is kept in a small clean stall. If infection is present, broad-spectrum systemic antibiotics should be administered for a period of 3 to 5 days peri-operatively. The bandage can be removed after 5 days, and then another bandage is applied and left in place for 5 days, if necessary.

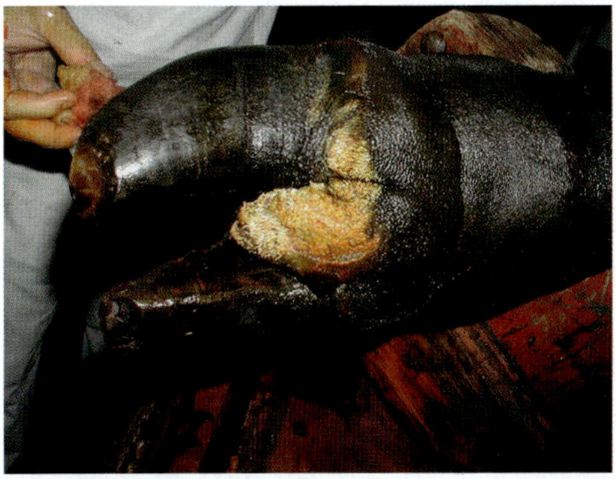

Fig. 17. Interdigital hyperplasia of the right hind foot. The growth is protruding dorsally.

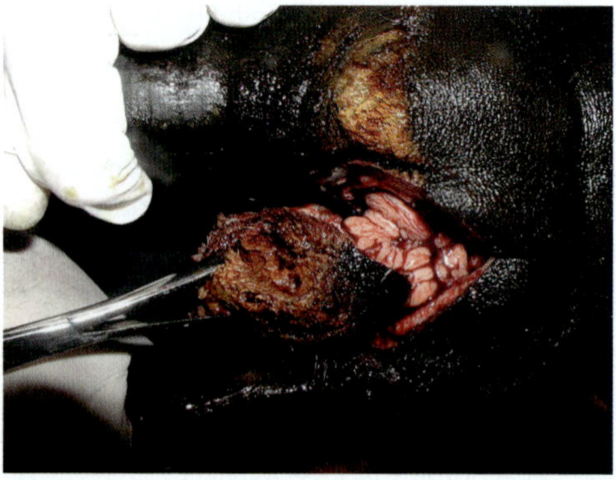

Fig. 18. The hyperplasia is grasp with a LaHey forceps to help the dissection. The interdigital fat can be seen underneath the growth.

VERTICAL FISSURES

Vertical fissures or sandcracks are linear and longitudinal defects of the dorsal claw wall. It is more common in beef breeds, with a prevalence up to 28%.[25,26] The front lateral digits are more commonly affected. The etiology of the fissures is unknown, although it is more common in older cattle. Fracture toughness and percentage of dehydration of the horn do not seem to affect vertical fissure formation.[27,28] The width of the fissure gradually increases as the animal get older, if not treated.[26]

In some cattle, the corion is exposed through the fissure, making the animal lame. When clinical signs are associated fissures, surgical debridement is advised. This can be done with the curve of a hoof knife or a motorized burr. Debridement should be done with care so as not to further traumatize the sensitive laminae. A 1-cm bar or triangle (1 cm at the base) may be used to make grooves at the end of the crack to redistribute the force and prevent further extension of the crack. Suture of the crack with wire also prevents the extension of the crack and decreases the pain engendered by movement of the wall on the sensitive laminae (**Fig. 19**). Holes are drilled 0.5-cm to 1-cm apart along the crack and an interrupted suture with wire or umbilical tape can be used. If the dermis is not infected, PMMA can be applied to fill the defect and the sutures are tied subsequently. In some cases, wire cannot be thread through the

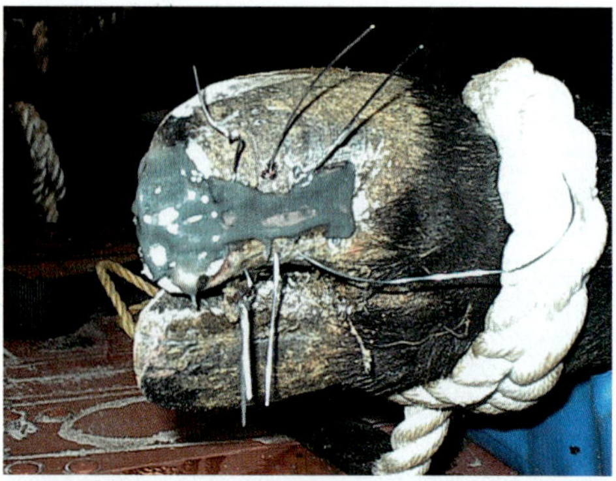

Fig. 19. After debridement of the vertical crack, wires are placed, the defect is filled with PMMA, and before it sets the wires are tightened.

damage hoof wall. Then, PMMA alone can be applied. If sensitive laminae are exposed or infection is present, PMMA application should be delayed until infection is controlled and the exposed laminae are covered with keratinized tissue. In severe cases, a wooden block should be applied on the healthy digit and the animal allowed to rest in a stall. The prognosis is good to excellent if the sensitive laminae are not infected. Supplemental dietary biotin was studied in a clinical trial on Hereford beef cows. Biotin (10 mg per head per day) in a free choice mineral supplement decreases the prevalence of vertical fissure of 50% over an 18-month period.[29]

SUMMARY

With a good knowledge of the anatomy of the foot and basic surgical instruments, digit surgery can be performed in a field situation. Sepsis of the DIP and PIP joint should be treated surgically because conservative treatment is often ineffective. Most of the diseases described in this article are chronic, and the animal has often been suffering for a while. Perioperative analgesia is very important to alleviate the pain of such animals. All procedures should be performed under local or regional anesthesia.

REFERENCES

1. Desrochers A, Anderson DE. Anatomy of the distal limb. Vet Clin North Am Food Anim Pract 2001;17:25–38.
2. Budras K, Habel RE. Bovine Anatomy. 1st edition. Hannover (Germany): Schlütersche; 2003. p. 138.
3. Fiedler A, Maierl J, Nuss K. Erkrankungen der Klauen und Zehen des Rindes. 1st edition. Stuttgart (Germany): Schattauer; 2004. p. 216 [in German].
4. Heppelmann M, Rehage J, Kofler J, et al. Ultrasonographic diagnosis of septic arthritis of the distal interphalangeal joint in cattle. Vet J, in press.
5. Greenough PR, Ferguson JG. Alternatives to amputation. Vet Clin North Am Food Anim Pract 1985;1:195–203.
6. Pejsa TG, St Jean G, Hoffsis GF, et al. Digit amputation in cattle: 85 cases (1971–1990). J Am Vet Med Assoc 1993;202:981–4.
7. Desrochers A, St Jean G. Surgical management of digit disorders in cattle. Vet Clin North Am Food Anim Pract 1996;12:277–98.
8. Funk KA. Late results of digit amputation in cattle. Berl Munch Tierartztl Wochenschr 1977;90:152–6.
9. Starke A. Resection of the distal interphalangeal joint and digital amputation in 21 breeding bulls: outcome and long-term follow-up. In: Nice (France): World Buiatric Congress; 2006.
10. Starke A, Heppelmann M, Beyerbach M, et al. Septic arthritis of the distal interphalangeal joint in cattle: comparison of digital amputation and joint resection by solar approach. Vet Surg 2007;36:350–9.
11. Bicalho RC, Cheong SH, Warnick LD, et al. The effect of digit amputation or arthrodesis surgery on culling and milk production in Holstein dairy cows. J Dairy Sci 2006;89:2596–602.
12. Nuss K. Surgery of the bovine digit. In: Anderson DE, Rings DM, editors. Current veterinary therapy 5, food animal practice. St. Louis (MO): Saunders Elsevier; 2009. p. 242–61.
13. Clemente CH. Contribution to the development of tendon resection and pedal joint resection in cattle. Tierärztl Umsch 1965;20:108–10.

14. Mulon P, Babkine M, d'Anjou MA, et al. Distal Interphalangeal joint degenerative disease in calves: a retrospective of 9 cases (1994–2004). In: San Diego (CA): American College of Veterinary Surgeons Veterinary Symposium; 2005. p. 18.
15. Kostlin RG, Nuss K. Treatment of the purulent hoof joint inflammation in cattle by joint resection-results. Tierarztl Prax 1998;16(2):123–31.
16. Bicalho RC, Cheong SH, Guard CL. Field technique for the resection of the distal interphalangeal joint and proximal resection of the deep digital flexor tendon in cows. Vet Rec 2007;160:435–9.
17. Greenough PR, MacCallum FJ, Weaver AD. Lameness in cattle. 2nd edition. Philadelphia: Lippincott; 1981.
18. Zulauf M, Jordan P, Steiner A. Fenestration of the abaxial hoof wall and implantation of gentamicin-impregnated collagen sponges for the treatment of septic arthritis of the distal interphalangeal joint in cattle. Vet Rec 2001;149:516–8.
19. Kofler J. Septic arthritis of the proximal interphalangeal (pastern) joint in cattle—clinical, radiographic, ultrasonographic findings and treatment. Berl Münch Tierärztl Wochenschr 1995;108:281–9.
20. Kofler J. Clinical study of toe ulcer and necrosis of the apex of the distal phalanx in 53 cattle. Vet J 1999;157:139–47.
21. Collick DW. Interdital hyperplasia. In: Greenough PR, editor. Lameness in Cattle. 3rd edition. Philadelphia: W.B. Sauders; 1997. p. 119–20.
22. Böttger T. Incidence of interdigital overgrowth in B and W bulls and its relationship to age. Dtsch Tierarztl Wochenschr 1962;69:596.
23. van Amstel SR, Shearer JK. Manual for treatment and control of lameness in cattle. 1st edition. Ames (IA): Blackwell Publishing; 2006. p. 212.
24. Holzhauer M, Bartels CJ, Dopfer D, et al. Clinical course of digital dermatitis lesions in an endemically infected herd without preventive herd strategies. Vet J 2008;177:222–30.
25. Goonewardene LA, Hand RK. A study of hoof cracks in grazing cattle; association of age, weight and fatness. Can J Anim Sci 1995;75:25–9.
26. Goonewardene LA, Hand RK, Wang S, et al. A study on the occurrence of sand cracks in commercial beef cattle. Journal of Animal and Veterinary Advances 2004;3:864–71.
27. Clark C, Petrie L. Fracture toughness of bovine claw horn from cattle with and without vertical fissures. Vet J 2007;173:541–7.
28. Clark CR, Petrie L, Waldner C, et al. Characteristics of the bovine claw associated with the presence of vertical fissures (sandcracks). Can Vet J 2004;45:585–93.
29. Campbell JR, Greenough PR, Petrie L. The effects of dietary biotin supplementation on vertical fissures of the claw wall in beef cattle. Can Vet J 2000;41:690–4.

Management of Tendon Disorders in Cattle

David E. Anderson, DVM, MS[a,*], André Desrochers, DMV, MS[b], Guy St. Jean, DMV, MS[c]

KEYWORDS

- Tendon • Congenital • Acquired • Laceration • Avulsion
- Tenosynovitis

Tendon disorders are a recognized cause of locomotory dysfunction in cattle, but the prevalence of lameness caused by tendon injury presently is unknown. Survey studies estimating the incidence of lameness in dairy herds in the United States, Canada, and the United Kingdom have not identified tendon disorders as a major cause of lameness.[1–3] However, one study indicated tendon involvement in 21% of limb lesions.[4] Another study reported that muscle or tendon lesions accounted for 74% of upper limb injuries in the forelimb and 7.8% in the hindlimb.[5] Tendon injuries causing loss of a production animal or a decreased level of production result in significant economic loss to the cattle producer. Tendon disorders may be congenital or acquired. Congenital abnormalities include lax tendons, contracted tendons, and displaced tendons. Acquired tendon disorders include lax tendons, contracted tendons, luxated tendons, tendinitis, lacerated tendons, avulsed tendons, ruptured tendons, and tenosynovitis.

CONGENITAL TENDON DISORDERS

Hyperextension Deformities

Flexor tendon laxity is generally the cause of hyperextension deformities in newborn calves. Such laxity occurs more commonly in calves born prematurely and in calves that are small for their gestational age. Acquired hyperextension deformities usually result from excessive weight-bearing caused by contralateral limb lameness or occur following removal of external coaptation after a prolonged period. Unilateral or bilateral hyperextension of the tarsus can be encountered in newborn calves following forced extraction. A rupture of the peroneus tertius causes the hyperextension of the tarsus. The gait is abnormal but it does not appear to be painful.

[a] Department of Clinical Sciences, College of Veterinary Medicine, Kansas State University, 1800 Denison Avenue, Manhattan, KS 66506, USA
[b] Department of Clinical Sciences, Université de Montréal, C.P. 5000 Saint-Hyacinthe, Quebec J2S 7C6, St-Hyacinthe, Quebec J2S 7C6, Canada
[c] Ross University School of Veterinary Medicine, P.O. Box 334, Basseterre, St-Kitts, West Indies
* Corresponding author.
E-mail address: danderso@vet.ksu.edu (D.E. Anderson).

Vet Clin Food Anim 24 (2008) 551–566
doi:10.1016/j.cvfa.2008.07.008 vetfood.theclinics.com
0749-0720/08/$ – see front matter © 2008 Elsevier Inc. All rights reserved.

Mild-to-moderate hyperextension commonly responds to limited exercise (myotactic reflex) that strengthens and tones the muscles, tendons, and ligaments. If exercise is not successful, some form of heel extension can be used to prevent hyperextension of the distal interphalangeal joint and keep the toe on the ground. The authors have used a thin wooden block glued to the hoof wall with methylmethacrylate acrylic (Technovit, Jorgensen Laboratories, Loveland, Colorado) to obtain heel extension. When methymethacrylate has to be used on calves' claws, the heat from the acrylic setting must be controlled by pouring cold water onto the surface of the acrylic. Otherwise the corium can be damaged.

Flexural Deformities

Flexural limb deformities occurring in a sagittal plane reflect an inability to achieve or maintain normal extension of the limb (**Fig. 1**).[6] Because flexural deformities often involve more than one structure, it is useful to describe them in terms of joints affected, rather than in terms of the affected tendons and ligaments. Congenital contracted flexor tendon is a common defect in cattle and occurs in numerous breeds.[7] Etiologic origins for contracted flexor tendons include inherited factors, in utero malpositioning, and overcrowding caused by the size of the fetus relative to the dam. Contracted tendons may occur with other congenital abnormalities, such as cleft palate, dwarfism, and arthrogryposis. A complete physical examination should be performed on the calf to rule out other problems before treatment is initiated for contracted tendons. Older cattle may acquire contracted tendons as a result of disease of the limb (eg, fracture or radial nerve paralysis, physitis).

The majority of contracted tendons in calves are observed within the first few days after birth. If one has reason to suspect a joint lesion as well as a tendinous lesion, radiographic examination may be useful before a prognosis is made and therapy is undertaken. Flexural deformities generally are found around the carpus or fetlock (**Fig. 2**). Flexural deformities are classified as mild (if the calves are able to walk on their feet but the heels do not contact the ground), moderate (if the dorsal aspect of the hoof breaks over a vertical plane perpendicular to the ground), or severe (if the affected animals are forced to walk on the dorsal aspect of the pastern, fetlock, or carpus). Often, nutrient or colostrum intake is not sufficient because the calves are unable to walk. Colostrum should be administered orally or plasma administered intravenously if the calf has difficulty walking. Also, unless adequate bedding is used or unless

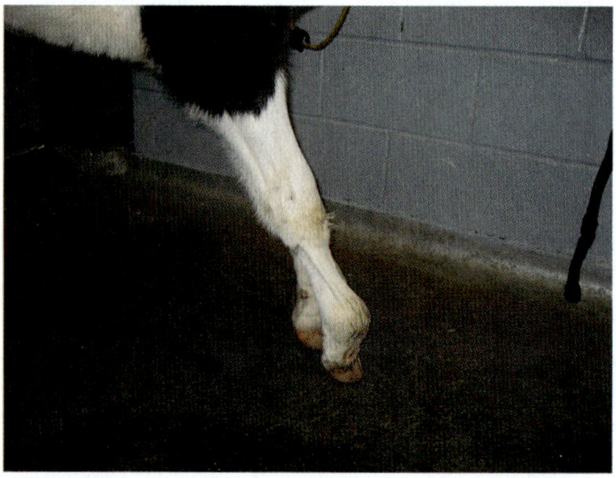

Fig. 1. Flexor tendon contracture in a Holstein calf causing hyperflexion of the metacarpophalangeal joints.

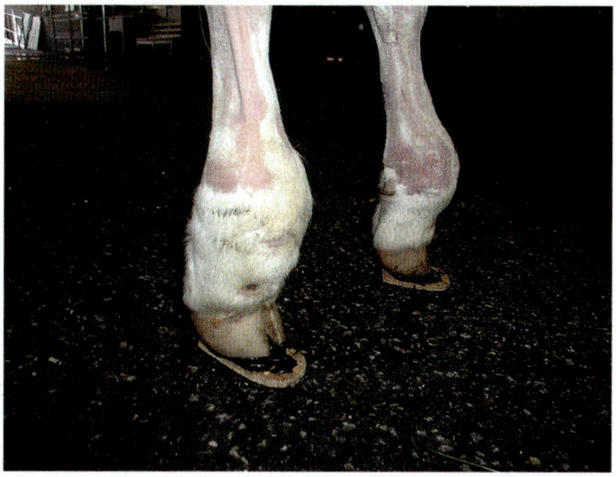

Fig. 2. Flexor tendon contracture causing hyperflexion of the metacarpophalangeal joints treated using an extended-toe block.

preventive measures are taken, rapid abrasion of the skin can occur from repeated trauma. Successful treatment of flexural deformities depends on the site and severity of the deformity and on the appropriate use of medical, physical, and possible surgical therapy. Treatment of congenital flexural deformities should be initiated soon after recognition of the problem, with the severity of the condition dictating how treatment should proceed. As the animal gets older, the contracted tissues become less responsive. Mild-to-moderate flexural deformities usually respond to physical therapy with manual stretching of the tendons during exercise. The authors commonly construct an extended toe shoe, using methylmethacrylate acrylic and a thin wooden block, to increase the tension on the contracted tendons during exercise (**Fig. 3**). Moderate cases are treated by using a bandage, splint, or cast and by providing analgesia using a nonsteroidal anti-inflammatory drug. Nonsteroidal anti-inflammatory drugs provide analgesia to the calf and are useful for decreasing the pain associated with the stretching of the contracted soft tissue caused by weight bearing, passive stretching exercise, splints, or casts. In one case, only one dose of oxytetracycline administered intravenously at 44 mg/kg was necessary for a short-term (96 hours), moderate decrease in the metacarpophalangeal joint angle of a newborn foal.[8] The mechanism by which oxytetracycline exerts its effect is unknown but it is most likely associated to a muscle relaxant effect.[8] To the authors' knowledge, the effect of oxytetracycline on contracted tendons in calves has not been studied scientifically. However, we do not recommend the routine use of oxytetracycline at this high dose in cattle because of the risk of inducing renal failure. A lower dose of tetracycline has been used to avoid renal failure with some success if treated early in the process of the disease.

A firm limb bandage can induce relaxation of a calf limb. This may be because of the supportive and protective effect on the muscles, tendons, and ligaments. Bandages should be placed over the entire limb, with the calf sedated and placed in lateral recumbency. The toes should be left unbandaged to support some weight and further stretch the tendons. Three layers of sheet cotton folded over provide adequate padding and support for young calves. This relaxation also can be accomplished by the constant tension or stretching (inverse myotactic reflex) produced by splints or casts in calves with moderate-to-severe contractual deformities. Daily or every other day splints can be changed and the leg examined. In the forelimb, a splint extending from the hoof to the elbow should be used. In a hindlimb, the splint is placed from the foot to the point of the hock. The splint should be placed on the palmar/plantar

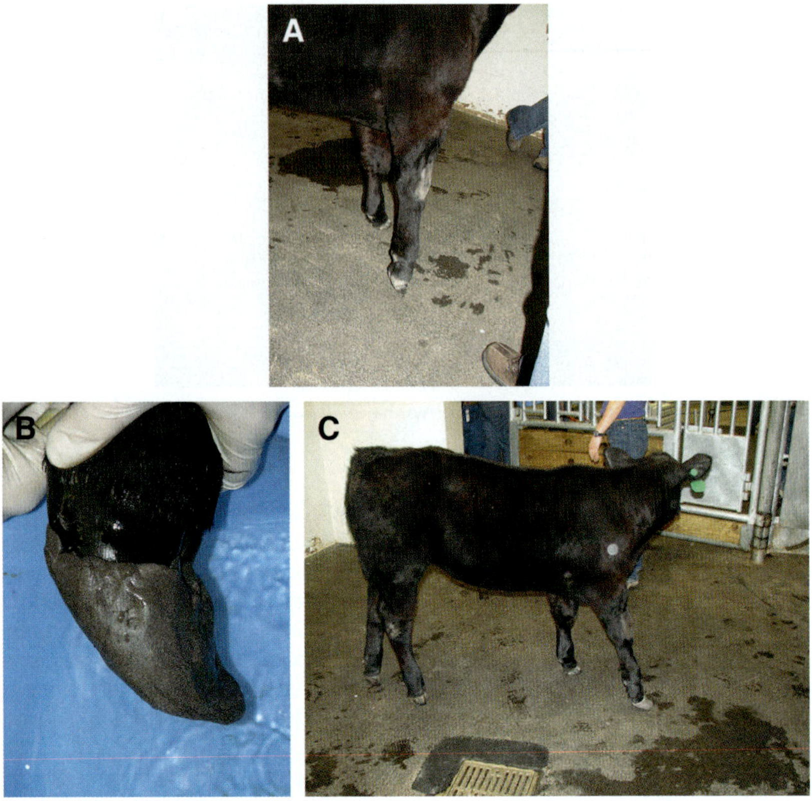

Fig. 3. (*A*) Calf with fetlock contracture caused by disuse of the limb during convalescence from a contralateral limb injury. (*B*) Hoof toe-extension created using polymethylmecralylate hoof cement. (*C*) Calf immediately after completion of application of an extended-toe shoe for treatment of fetlock contracture.

aspect of the limb. The splint can be fashioned from polyvinylchloride (PVC) pipe cut into a semitubular shape and should be padded well to avoid pressure sores. Splints can cause severe pressure sores and thus must be carefully monitored.

A cast may be necessary to provide more support, especially for calves with carpal flexural deformity. With the calf sedated and in lateral recumbency, a fiberglass cast is applied and allowed to harden as someone reduces the contracted limb into as normal a position as possible. The toes of the limb should be exposed so that the calf walks on the toes rather than on the cast. The cast should be removed in 1 week so that the limb can be examined. The cast can be reused as a bi-halved splint if necessary. The relaxation effect of bandages, splints, and casts often provides enough improvement to allow further gradual improvement with exercise.

Most flexural limb deformities correct with persistent nonsurgical management. Those that do not improve may benefit from surgery, but the results in severely contracted limbs are often disappointing, and these animals usually are sent to slaughter when they reach an acceptable weight. Calves with severe flexural deformities of the fetlock may be treated by tenotomy performed in the midmetacarpal or midmetatarsal region (**Fig. 4**) or proximal to the carpus if the carpus also is affected by a flexural deformity. With the animal anesthetized, all tendinous tissues under tension are severed

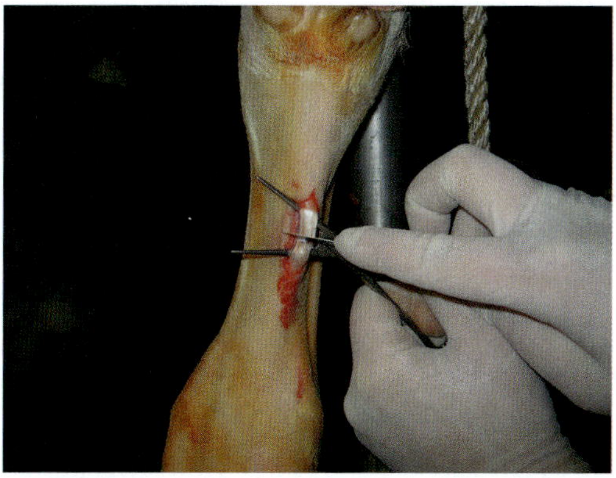

Fig. 4. Midmetacarpal flexor tenotomy for treatment of unresponsive fetlock contracture.

through a small incision until the limb can be fully extended. If the tenotomy results in some relief, but complete extension of the limb is still impossible, severe trauma to the periarticular tissues may be necessary to achieve adequate extension of the affected limbs. Bandaging and splinting of the limb for 1 to 2 weeks might be required postoperatively. If excessive relaxation of the limb is obtained, the limb, including the foot, should be placed in a cast for 3 to 4 weeks until the tendons are reunited by fibroplasia.

Arthrogryposis

Congenital arthrogryposis is defined as a syndrome of persistent joint contracture present at birth. Arthrogryposis may afflict one leg, the hind or front legs,[9] or all four legs, and has been reported in many breeds of cattle.[7] Arthrogryposis includes more than one etiologic and pathologic entity. A hereditary congenital deformity in Hereford cattle characterized by arthrogryposis, kyphosis, torticollis, scoliosis, and cleft palate has been described. Teratogens indentified as causing arthrogryposis include plants and prenatal viral infections. Ingestion of lupines by pregnant cows between 40 and 70 days' gestation has caused various degrees of arthrogryposis with other associated congenital defects.[10] Lupine toxicosis is related to high alkaloid content.[11]

Arthrogryposis should not be confused with contracted tendons in which the joints are aligned properly and the legs are not rotated. Usually, joints of calves with contracted tendons can be extended with pressure or corrected surgically. In calves with arthrogryposis and crooked calf disease, the articular and osseous changes usually are permanent and become worse as the calf grows. In one retrospective study on arthrogryposis including 113 calves, 74% of the animals had only the forelimbs (carpus and fetlock) contracted; in 75% of cases, a cesarean section was needed because of dystocia.[10] Predisposing factors to arthrogryposis were male gender, posterior intrauterine presentation, and double muscling. If untreated, arthrogryposis of the carpus usually is lethal in cattle. It usually results in skin necrosis over the carpus, septic arthritis, and septicemia. Surgical treatment is attempted to improve the animal's posture sufficiently for it to obtain slaughter weight.

Surgical treatment for arthrogryposis of the forelimbs has been published and consists of desmotomy and tenotomy of contracted penarticular soft tissues.[9,10] Often, all structures on the palmar aspect of the carpus, except blood vessels and nerves, are transected. A cast is then applied for a minimum of 6 weeks.

Approximately 80% of these surgically treated animals can be kept until they reach normal slaughter weight. Because of a possible hereditary component, the authors do not recommend keeping these animals for breeding. When palmar carpal ligament transection has been performed, carpal hyperextension may occur in the postoperative period. If the palmar angulation between the metacarpus and radius is less than 100° before surgery, the prognosis is poor. In these cases, arthrodesis of the carpus may be attempted.[10]

Spastic Paresis

Spastic paresis is a progressive neuromuscular disease that occurs in dairy, beef, and crossbred cattle. Signs of spastic paresis usually appear at a few weeks to several months of age.[11] Spastic contractions of one or both gastrocnemius muscles and superficial digital flexor (SDF) tendons lead to hyperextension of the hock. The affected leg is extended caudally and is advanced in a swinging motion. With progression of the disease, the foot often may not touch the ground, and gluteal muscle atrophy occurs. Palpation of the limb shows that the gastrocnemius muscle is hard and rigid, but flexion of the hock is not painful. The base of the tail often is elevated.

Initially, few if any systemic effects result from the condition. With its progression, however, the animal may remain recumbent for a longer period and lose weight. Calves often must be slaughtered prematurely. No consistent pathologic lesion has been identified in the peripheral musculature or nerves or in the spinal cord or brain of animals with spastic paresis. The functional disturbance may be due to an overactive stretch reflex present in the gastrocnemius muscles caused by overstimulation or lack of inhibition of motor neurons. Because spastic paresis is probably inherited to some degree, affected animals should not be used as breeding stock. Surgical treatment of spastic paresis may be indicated in selected animals, mostly either to allow the cattle to reach slaughter weight or to keep an animal for sentimental value. We recommend mandatory castration before surgical treatment of calves affected with spastic paresis.

Two techniques for correcting spastic paresis have been described: tibial neurectomy or transection of a portion of the gastrocnemius and SDF tendons.[12,13] Partial or complete tibial neurectomy is aesthetically more pleasing. The procedure can be performed under sedation and epidural anesthesia or under general anesthesia with the animal placed in lateral recumbency with the affected leg uppermost. The tibial nerve is found via a lateral incision through the biceps femoris muscle. The tibial nerve is located caudal to the peroneal nerve. The tibial nerve is isolated and its different branches are stimulated electrically to evaluate the corresponding muscle contraction. A 3-cm long segment is excised from each of the two nerve branches to the gastrocnemius. Closure is routine. Only one leg should be operated on at a time to assess the efficacy of the procedure. Partial tibial neurectomy has resulted in good-to-excellent results in 131 of 138 (95%) calves.[12] The authors have performed complete and partial tibial neurectomy on a large number of calves affected by spastic paresis. Although clinical improvement is obvious, the results are suboptimal, temporary (usually lasting 4 to 6 months), and often do not allow the calf to return to a level of productive performance intended by the owner. The expense of this procedure makes tibial neurectomy impractical.

Transection of a portion of the gastrocnemius and SDF tendons is performed after sedation, with the animal placed in lateral recumbency and with the affected leg uppermost.[13] The leg is surgically prepared from the midmetatarsus to the stifle and 2% lidocaine is locally infiltrated over a 10-cm length proximal to the calcaneus and over the cranial border of the lateral aspect of the calcaneal tendon. The two tendons of insertion of the gastrocnemius muscle (lateral and medial head of the gastrocnemius muscle) and half of the SDF tendons are transected for a length of 2 cm, approximately 6 cm proximal to the point of the hock. The subcutis is closed with a simple continuous pattern, followed by a layer of simple uninterrupted skin sutures of nonabsorbable monofilament material. A bandage is applied over the surgical site for 5 days, and the skin sutures are removed after 14 days. The immediate effect of surgery is that the hock becomes profoundly flexed and the metatarsus becomes nearly parallel to the ground. Fibrous unions generally develop between the tendon ends, and limb posture returns in 4 to 6 weeks. Spasticity often returns slowly over several months. The authors have performed complete or partial gastrocnemius tenotomy on a large number of calves. Although clinical improvement is obvious, the results are temporary, usually lasting 4 to 6 months, and often do not allow the calf to return to a level of productive performance expected by the owner. This procedure can easily be done in field conditions and may be preferred over tibial neurectomy because of the lower expense associated with the procedure.

ACQUIRED TENDON DISORDERS

Dairy breeds, feedlot cattle, and cattle maintained in confinement housing are commonly affected by acquired tendon disorders, and the incidence of lameness in dairy herds ranges widely. Lesions in dairy cattle occur most frequently during the early lactational period and in first-lactation heifers. Lesions may occur more frequently during the spring and summer. However, lameness caused by tendon injury seems uncommon in cattle. Because such injuries are less common, information regarding acquired tendon disorders in ruminants is limited. Injuries observed in cattle include tendon displacement, traumatic tendinitis, septic tenosynovitis, and tendon laceration, avulsion, or spontaneous rupture.

Septic Tendinitis

Septic tendinitis is most commonly associated with extension of digital sepsis, subsolar abscess, or sole ulcer (pododermatitis circumscripta, Rusterholz ulcer) to involve the deep digital flexor (DDF) tendon.[14,15] Avulsion of the DDF from its insertion on the flexor tuberosity of the distal phalanx (P3) may result if sufficient necrosis of the tendon or underlying bone occurs. Septic tendinitis also may occur when degloving injuries involve the flexor or extensor tendons of the distal limbs. Degloving wounds are often associated with injury from wire fencing, farm machinery, metal siding on buildings, trailer accidents, and dog attacks. Treatment includes thorough surgical debridement, lavage, daily wound management, and systemic antibiotic and anti-inflammatory medication. Antibiotic selection should be based on results of microbial culture and sensitivity. In the authors' experience, *Arcanobacterium pyogenes, Escherichia coli, Bacteroides* spp, and *Bacteriaceae* are the most commonly involved bacteria. For empiric therapy, procaine penicillin G (22,000 U/kg, intramuscularly [IM] or subcutaneously [SC], every 24 hours), sodium ceftiofur (2.2 mg/kg, IM, every 24 hours), or ampicillin trihydrate (10 to 22 mg/kg, IM/SC, every 24 hours) are the antibiotic treatments of choice when microbial cultures are not performed. If DDF tendon involvement is confined to a single digit, a wooden or rubber block (claw block) may be applied to the solar surface of the healthy digit to improve comfort and ambulation. We recommend that these animals be maintained in a restricted environment (stall or small pen) during convalescence (6 to 8 weeks). Also, the claw block should be removed before the animal is turned out to pasture to prevent damage to the tendons and ligaments of the healthy digit.

Prognosis for septic tendinitis is good for superficial wounds. Deep wounds causing extensive tissue necrosis or sepsis of adjacent synovial cavities (joints, tendon sheaths) warrant a more guarded prognosis.

Tendon Laceration

Tendon laceration is an uncommon cause of lameness in cattle and occurs most commonly when the cow falls onto or kicks a sharp object. The rear limbs are affected most commonly.[16] Typically an open wound with contamination or infection is present at the site of tendon rupture. Management practices may be associated with the higher incidence of tendon lacerations among dairy breeds. Adult dairy cattle are maintained in a high-concentration environment and are often moved on concrete flooring. Concrete flooring requires frequent cleaning, which is often done using a tractor with a blade attachment. Therefore, dairy cattle are exposed to potential hazards on the farm. Feedlot cattle are also housed in concentrated environments with frequent exposure to farm machinery. However, feedlot cattle may be infrequently presented for treatment because of their lower perceived individual economic value.

Lacerations occur most commonly in a single hindlimb at the level of the midmetatarsus. Ultrasound examination of the involved tissues may be limited because of the pressure of an open wound and emphysema of the peritendinous tissues.[17,18] Radiographs (survey, contrast studies) may be useful to determine if a joint or tendon sheath is involved and to evaluate for the presence of a foreign body.

Tendon Avulsion

In our experience, the most common tendon avulsion of cattle is avulsion of the DDF tendon from its insertion on the solar aspect of the third phalanx. Avulsion of the DDF tendon usually occurs secondary to sepsis of P3 and necrosis of the tendon insertion caused by subsolar abscess, sole ulcer, septic arthritis of the distal interphalangeal joint, or septic pedal osteitis.[19] We also have observed avulsion of the calcaneal tendon from its insertion on the calcaneus secondary to septic apophysitis in calves. Septic apophysitis was presumably caused by hematogenous bacterial colonization. We also have diagnosed several animals affected with avulsion of the gastrocnemius muscle from its origin on the distal caudal femur. Traumatic tendon avulsion affecting the peroneus tertius muscle has occurred in calves immediately after removal of a full-limb cast. We have seen traumatic avulsion of the tendon of insertion of the extensor carpi radialis muscle in a calf after manual extraction for treatment of dystocia.

Management should be directed toward support of the limb and treatment of the inciting disease. Treatment may include stall rest and anti-inflammatory medication. Surgical debridement, lavage, and daily wound management is indicated for deep sole ulcer, subsolar abscess, and septic pedal osteitis. Because a septic process is often at the origin of the avulsion of the DDF tendon from the distal phalanx, a facilitated ankylosis of the distal interphalangeal joint is favored to stabilize the foot. Affected cattle should be confined to a small pen or a stall for 6 to 8 weeks. The prognosis for uniaxial DDF tendon avulsion is good if the cause of infection is treated.

A full-limb cast was used to treat a calf with avulsion of the tendon of insertion of the extensor carpi radialis muscle. The cast was removed after 21 days, and stall rest continued for 14 days. The calf made a full recovery, without complications. Avulsion of the gastrocnemius muscle may be treated using a Thomas splint to stabilize the limb, but a poor prognosis for return to productive soundness should be given for complete avulsion. Stall rest for 8 to 12 weeks is recommended for partial gastrocnemius muscle avulsion. The owner should receive a guarded to fair prognosis for the animal.

Tendon Rupture

Spontaneous tendon rupture is most commonly associated with breeding accidents, bull fights, or postpartunent neuropathy and usually involves the gastrocnemius muscle-tendon unit. Spontaneous rupture of the gastrocnemius muscle usually occurs at the junction of the muscle fibers and tendon (**Fig. 5**).[16,20–23] Direct trauma may cause rupture of the gastrocnemius tendon adjacent to the insertion on the tuber calcaneus. Flexor tendon rupture may occur secondary to septic tendinitis, necrosis, and sepsis of peritendinous tissues. Septic tendinitis often occurs from open wounds or degloving injuries. Also, rupture of the DDF tendon may occur secondary to septic pedal osteitis, septic arthritis of the distal interphalangeal joint, or septic flexor tenosynovitis.[14]

Treatment of Tendon Disruption

Flexor tendon lacerations can be managed successfully in cattle by tenorrhaphy and external coaptation or by external coaptation alone. Economic costs associated with treatment and prolonged convalescence should be discussed with the owner before attempting therapy. Also, the owner's expectation for long-term productivity should include the likelihood of persistent lameness.

Options for treatment of tendon laceration in cattle include stall rest, use of a wooden or rubber block on the healthy digit, cast application, tenorrhaphy, and corrective farriery (**Fig. 6**). The location of the lesion, individual tendon involvement, and concurrent injuries are important factors for treatment selection.[24] Stall confinement may be adequate for incomplete lacerations and partial disruption of the gastrocnemius muscle or tendon. Application of a wooden block is useful when the branches of the DDF tendons (III or IV) to a single digit are disrupted. A full-limb or half-limb cast may be indicated for injuries disrupting the flexor tendons to both digits of the same limb. Stall rest, use of a wooden block, and external coaptation of the limb result in healing of the tendon by second intention (fibroplasia) and scar tissue formation. Flexor tendon laceration located distal to the hock may be treated with application of a cast that includes the foot and extends to the level of the hock but does not

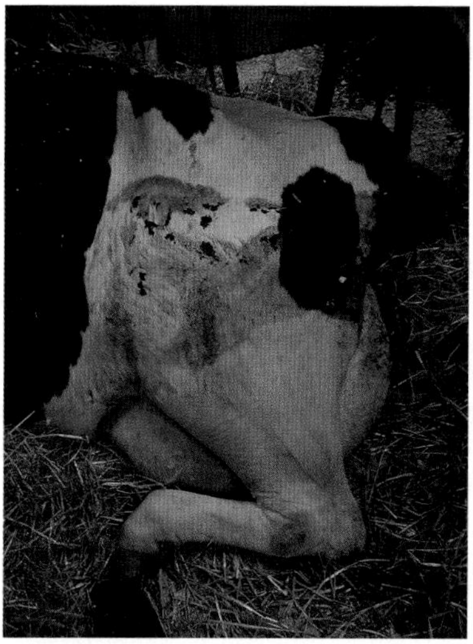

Fig. 5. Simultaneous flexion of hock and extension of stifle in a recumbent cow suffering avulsion of the gastrocnemius muscle from its origin on the femur.

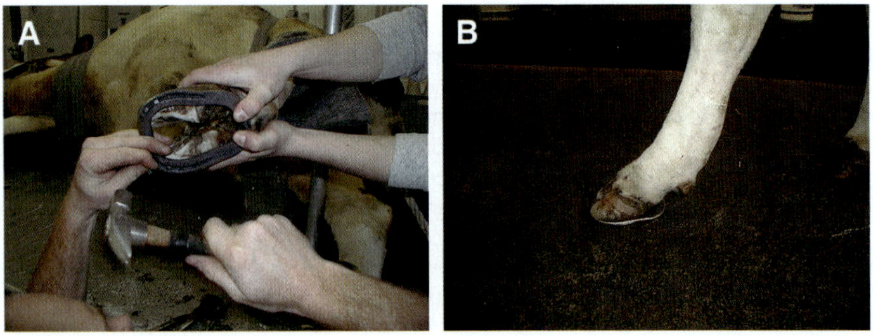

Fig. 6. (*A*) Use of corrective farriery to treat flexor tendon laxity. The corrective shoe being nailed onto the hoof has an extended heel component. (*B*) Posture of calf standing with corrective shoe. The heel extension from the shoe supports the fetlock while simultaneously keeping the sole and toe region of the digits in contact with the ground.

span the hock.[25,26] The fetlock may be flexed during casting to release tension from the tendons and allow closer apposition of the tendon ends. Alternatively, the limb may be cast in a normal, standing position. We recommend that the cast be maintained for 3 to 4 weeks longer than when a "flexed fetlock" cast is used. The fetlock must be lightly padded on the dorsal and palmar/plantar aspect to protect the limb from pressure-induced cast sores (ulcerations). Laceration of the calcaneal tendon may be treated with application of a cast that includes the foot and extends to the proximal tibia (level of the tibial crest). The portion of the cast spanning the hock must be thicker than the remainder of the cast to prevent the cast from breaking at this point. Reinforcing splints may provide a stronger structure and, if used, should be placed on the tension and compression sides of the limb. Thomas splints may be used to stabilize gastrocnemius muscle-tendon disruption. However, in our experience, the results have been poor. We prefer to use a full-limb cast when the disruption is close to the calcaneus.

Suture repair (tenorrhaphy) of transected tendons in addition to external coaptation achieves a more mature scar and a stronger scar-tendon unit more rapidly than does healing by second intention. The surgeon should have a good working knowledge of limbanectomy.[27,28] Biomechanical tests of the various methods of tenorrhaphy have resulted in the recommendation that double– or triple–interlocking-loop or three-loop pulley suture patterns be used. The SDF tendon, DDF tendon, and suspensory ligament divide distally in cattle to provide one main branch to each digit. The bodies of the tendons in the metacarpal and metatarsal regions are wide and thin and present a challenge for anchorage of tendon sutures. In our clinical experience, the three-loop pulley suture pattern provides superior suture-holding power in damaged flexor tendons of cattle. However, we have not observed a clinically significant advantage using tenorrhaphy and external coaptation compared with external coaptation alone. Subtle benefits of tenorrhaphy may not be observed in cattle because they are not required to perform maximal exercise. Nylon, polydioxanon, and polyglyconate are the most common suture material used for tendon repair. However, no suture material nor any suture pattern currently in use can provide adequate breaking strength to allow ambulation without external coaptation. In horses, normal flexor tendons endure strain of approximately 5% when walking (without a rider).

Cast immobilization has been advocated for a minimum of 4 to 5 weeks based on biomechanical studies of tendon healing and on clinical observations. Supportive farriery also has been recommended after cast removal. Currently, the authors recommend external coaptation be maintained for a minimum of 60 days after complete transection of flexor tendons. After cast removal, a block may be used to elevate the heel and stall confinement should be continued for 2 to 4 weeks after cast removal. Elevation of the heel in the range of 40° to 70° decreases tendon strain in the DDF tendon but not in the SDF tendon or the suspensory ligament in horses. Heel elevation after cast removal is not required when a "standing conformation" cast has been used.

The prognosis for tendon rupture in cattle is considered good for injuries involving the SDF tendon alone. In our experience, the prognosis for survival and for long-term productivity of cattle with traumatic rupture of the digital flexor tendons (SDF DDF, suspensory ligament) is fair to good. Ultrasound examination of the healing tendon may provide valuable information regarding treatment and prognosis. Treatment of gastrocnemius tendon rupture has only been recommended for young, lightweight cattle. In cases of complete disruption of the calcaneal tendon or gastrocnemius muscle, we provide a grave prognosis for cattle weighing more than 500 kg, and a poor prognosis for cattle weighing less than 500 kg. The prognosis for production soundness after disruption of the extensor tendons is considered excellent.

TENOSYNOVITIS (TENOVAGINITIS)

Based on research reported for horses, the tendon sheath has a structure that is distinctly different from that of diarthroidal joints. The synovial lining cells of the tendon sheath are fibroblastic in appearance and are composed of a single synovial cell type (diarthroidal joints have two distinct cell types).[29] Also, the tendon sheath contains abundant blood vessels but few nerve fibers. Synovial fluid produced by the tendon sheath has a lower concentration of hyaluronic acid and a lower mucinous precipitate quality than those of diarthroidal joint fluid. However, the cellular constituents and protein concentration in tendon sheath fluid and joint fluid are similar. Cellular and protein changes in response to trauma and sepsis are also similar.

Pathologic lesions occur most commonly in the digital flexor tendon sheath. Staneck[30] reported a that 10.7% of 766 cattle hospitalized suffered from tenosynovitis. The digital flexor tendon sheath originates from a point 6 to 8 cm proximal to the fetlock and extends distally to a point immediately distal to the coronary band. The tendon sheath is confined on its palmar/plantar surface by the palmar/plantar annular ligament of the fetlock, the palmar/plantar digital annular ligament (distal to the accessory digits or dewclaw), and the distal interdigital ligaments (proximal to the heel bulbs). Inflammation of the digital tendon sheath should be suspected when focal swelling of the palmar/plantar aspect of the pastern is observed concurrent with focal swelling extending proximally from the level of the dewclaws.

Inflammation of synovial structures may be caused by trauma, injection of irritant chemicals, immune-mediated synovitis, or sepsis. Inflammation and distension of the tendon sheath result in pain.[30,31] Adhesions between the tendon and tendon sheath may result from sustained trauma or inflammation. Restrictive adhesions may cause recurrent pain and lead to decreased productive soundness. Two forms of tenosynovitis have been recognized in cattle: aseptic (traumatic, secondary synovitis, idiopathic) and septic (direct extension, iatrogenic, hematogenous). The authors have successfully treated various cattle affected with aseptic tenosynovitis using nonsteroidal anti-inflammatory drugs, warm-water hydrotherapy (30 minutes, two to three times per day for 10 to 14 days), tendon sheath drainage and lavage (1-L 0.9% saline or lactated Ringer's solution, once), pressure bandages (changed every 2 days for 7 to

10 days), and/or intrathecal sodium hyaluronate (20 mg, once).[32–36] Selection of treatment is based on severity, location of the involved tendon sheath, and economic constraints.

Septic Tenosynovitis

Septic tenosynovitis is most frequently diagnosed in the digital flexor tendon sheath but also commonly occurs in the tendon sheath of the extensor carpi radialis muscle. Sepsis of the tendon sheath typically occurs as a result of extension of local sepsis (such as with sole ulcer, a septic distal interphalangeal joint, a septic navicular bursa or podotrochleosis, or a heel bulb abscess) or by direct inoculation (via penetrating wounds, foreign bodies, or iatrogenic trauma from farm implements, such as a pitchfork or front-end loader).[14–16] Septic tenosynovitis caused by hematogenous translocation of bacteria (septicemia) is rare. Clinical signs include lameness (moderate to non–weight-bearing), recumbency, decreased milk production, and decreased feed intake. When standing, affected cattle may be reluctant to walk or may walk with the limb abducted or adducted to shift weight to the unaffected digit. Purulent effusion of the tendon sheath results in swelling proximal to the accessory digits (dewclaws). Swelling in the pastern region is limited by the annular ligament of the fetlock, the digital annular ligament, and the proximal interdigital ligaments. The lateral portion of the hindlimb tendon sheath is more frequently affected. Diagnosis of septic tenosynovitis may include physical examination, synovial fluid collection for cytologic evaluation and culture, and radiography. Insertion of a blunt probe through the wound or injection of contrast material into the wound may facilitate diagnosis of septic tenosynovitis.

Treatment of septic tenosynovitis should include management of the inciting disease and of the infected tendon sheath. Each digital branch of the DDF tendon has its own tendon sheath, but the two sheaths communicate near their proximal extent. Interestingly, septic tenosynovitis does not commonly occur in both tendon sheaths concurrently. The excessive fibrinous response to intrathecal sepsis, typical of cattle, may serve to localize infection to a single digital tendon sheath. Medical management alone (systemic antibiotics, hydrotherapy, protective bandages) is unlikely to be effective because of the severity of the inciting disease and the excessive fibrin deposition within the tendon sheath. This relationship was demonstrated for septic arthritis in cattle when medical treatment successfully resolved the infection in 43% of affected cattle and surgical treatment resolved the infection in 73% of affected cattle. Antibiotics cannot effectively penetrate fibrin foci to achieve therapeutic concentrations.[6,7] Effective treatment of septic tenosynovitis involves surgical debridement and lavage of the affected tendon sheath (in valuable breeding animals) or digit amputation (in commercial cattle or cattle intended for salvage).

Several techniques may be used for surgical debridement, drainage, and lavage of the tendon sheath. Surgical exploration of the tendon sheath provides optimal access for thorough debridement of the tendon sheath and tendon. Exploration is performed by incising the sheath beginning at its origin proximal to the accessory digits and extending distally to a point approximately 2 cm proximal to the coronary band. After debridement and lavage of the sheath, the sheath may be closed primarily or an indwelling Penrose drain, exiting proximally and distally, may be used to facilitate drainage after surgery. The Penrose drain is removed approximately 5 days after surgery and a bandage is maintained for an additional 5 days after the drain is removed. However, this technique is associated with extensive tissue damage and risk of injury to the neurovascular supply to the distal limb. Dehiscence of the surgical wound is another potential complication because of the high motion occurring in the palmar/plantar aspect of the fetlock. We do not recommend this technique for routine use. The tendon sheath is better left open if the tendons are necrotic and had to be resected.

In our experience, the treatment of choice for septic tenosynovitis without the necrotic tendinitis in cattle is surgical implantation of an active lavage system using a multifenestrated silicone rubber drain (Snyder Hemovac, Zimmer, Dover, Ohio). This procedure is best performed with the animal sedated and restrained in lateral recumbency on a tilt table. Intravenous regional anesthesia (lidocaine 2%, 20 mL) is infused distal to a tourniquet before surgery. We routinely administer sodium or potassium penicillin (1 million units) distal to the tourniquet after the anesthetic has been instilled. Before surgery, a wooden block is applied to the healthy digit to improve comfort and ambulation during the convalescent period. A needle is inserted in the tendon sheath to verify correct location. A 14-gauge needle is inserted into the tendon sheath proximally and distally to guide optimal placement of the stab incisions. Then, limited debridement is performed through a stab incision placed into the proximal aspect of the tendon sheath and a second stab incision placed into the distal tendon sheath. A large, curved forceps or clamp (Rochester-Carmalt forceps) is inserted from proximal to distal within the tendon sheath. The instrument is used to grasp the proximal tubing of the drain, and the drain is pulled through the tendon sheath. The drain is then sutured into place and the excess fenestrated portion of the drain is discarded. Drainage and lavage is performed by high-pressure infusion of sterile, isotonic electrolyte solutions into the drain and by allowing the fluid to exit distally around the end of the drain. We use a 60-mL syringe and three-way stopcock to achieve high-pressure lavage. The distal end of the drain is sutured closed to occlude the lumen and force the fluids to exit the drain into the tendon sheath. The drain is sutured to the skin proximally and distally and maintained under a sterile bandage between flushing. High-pressure lavage is performed once daily for 5 to 7 days, using 1 to 2 L of saline or lactated Ringer's solution. Crystalline antibiotic solutions may be instilled into the drain and tendon sheath after each lavage or when the drain is removed. Many veterinarians add antiseptic chemicals (such as povidone iodine or chlorhexidine) to lavage fluids. However, research has shown that povidone iodine (concentration >0.2%) and chlorhexidine (concentration >0.05%) induce significant synovitis[37–39] and may exacerbate intrathecal disease. No significant benefit was observed with use of 0.1% povidone iodine solution based on bacterial cultures and histologic evaluation in in vivo experimental models of septic arthritis in horses.

Optimally, the drain should be cultured at the time of removal and the results compared with initial microbial cultures. Systemic antibiotics and anti-inflammatory medication are administered concurrently. Ascending infection of the tendon sheath is a possible complication with this technique. Also, higher costs associated with placement of the lavage system and daily wound and bandage management limit the use of this technique. In our experience, a good-to-excellent prognosis for long-term productive soundness may be given with this technique.

Digit amputation proximal to the middle phalanx provides ventral drainage of purulent material and fibrin from the tendon sheath. Immediate relief from pain and swelling may be noted after surgery. Antibiotics should be administered for 7 to 10 days after surgery, but may be omitted if early salvage is performed. This treatment limits the productive longevity of the animal.

Antibiotic and Anti-Inflammatory Therapy

Treatment of cattle with antibiotic or anti-inflammatory drugs must be instituted with consideration for potential drug efficacy, toxicity, and residues. Many drugs commonly used in food animal practice are used at extralabel doses, routes, volumes per injection site, and frequency. The veterinarian is compelled to follow strict guidelines (veterinarian–client–patient relationship) when electing to use extralabel drugs. The reader is referred to pharmacology texts and proper regulatory agencies for policies regarding the extralabel use of drugs and proper withdrawal times for meat and milk to avoid residue violations.

Optimally, selection of an appropriate antibiotic is based on in vitro microbial culture and sensitivity results. However, culturing bacteria from synovial fluid is often difficult. Therefore, empiric antibiotic selection may be elected when culture results are negative or because of economic constraints. When empiric therapy is chosen, antibiotic selection should be based on known, common pathogens involved in deep tissue sepsis in cattle and on antibiotics known to achieve adequate tissue distribution. Common pathogens isolated from septic musculoskeletal lesions in cattle include *A pyogenes, Streptococcus* spp, *Staphylococcus* spp, *Fusobacterium necrophorum, Bacteroides* spp, and coliforms.[40,41] In the authors' experience, the most common pathogens involved in septic arthritis and tenosynovitis in adult cattle are *A pyogenes* and *E coli.* Antibiotics of choice include penicillin, cephalosporins, oxytetracycline, and trimethoprim-sulfa combinations (age dependent). Extralabel use of fluoroquinolone antibiotics has been banned by the Food and Drug Administration (Center for Veterinary Medicine).

The authors routinely use intra-articular or regional intravenous antibiotic infusions distal to a tourniquet as an adjunct treatment for sepsis of deep tissues (for example, distal interphalangeal joint sepsis, tenosynovitis, or septic cellulitis of the distal limb). This technique is used to achieve high concentrations of antibiotics in synovial spaces or peripheral tissues. Crystalline antibiotic solutions may be infused immediately after performing local intravenous regional anesthesia. Limited scientific research is available on this practice in veterinary medicine. Recently, the serum and synovial fluid pharmacokinetics after a single dose of cefazolin were reported for cattle.[42] Peak synovial fluid concentrations were achieved 30 to 90 minutes after antibiotic infusion. Currently, the authors maintain the tourniquet for 30 to 45 minutes after antibiotic infusion.

REFERENCES

1. Choquette-Levy L, Baril I, Levy M, et al. A study of foot disease of dairy cattle in Quebec. Can Vet J 1985;26:278–81.
2. Wells SJ, Trent AM, Marsh WE, et al. Prevalence and severity of lameness in lactating dairy cows in a sample of Minnesota and Wisconsin herds. J Am Vet Med Assoc 1993;02:78–82.
3. Whitaker DA, Kelly JM, Smith EJ. Incidence of lameness in dairy cows. Vet Rec 1983;13:60–2.
4. Russell AM, Rowlands GJ, Shaw SR, et al. Survey of lameness in British dairy cattle. Vet Rec 1982;111:155–60.
5. Arkins S. Lameness in dairy cows. Irish Vet J 1981;35:135–40.
6. Tulleniers EP. Management of bovine orthopedic problems, part II: coxofemoral luxation, soft tissue problems, sepsis, and miscellaneous skull problems. Compend Cont Educ Pract Vet 1986;8:5117–23.
7. Leipold HW, Hirarga T, Dennis SM. Congenital defects of the bovine musculoskeletal system and joints. Vet Clin North Am Food Anim Pract 1993;9:93–104.
8. Madison JB, Garber JL, Rice B, et al. Effect of oxytetracycline on metacarpophalangeal and distal interphalangeal joint angles in newborn foals. J Am Vet Med Assoc 1994;204:246–9.

9. Verschooten F, DeMoor A, Desmet P, et al. Surgical treatment of congenital arthrogryposis of the carpal joint associated with contraction of the flexor tendons in calves. Vet Rec 1969;85:140–71.
10. Van Huffel X, DeMoor A. Congenital multiple arthrogryposis of the forelimb in calves. Compend Cont Educ Pract Vet 1987;9(10):F333–9.
11. Leipold HW, Huston K, Guffy MM, et al. Spastic paresis in beef shorthorn cattle. J Am Vet Med Assoc 1967;151:598–601.
12. Vlaminck L, De Moor A, Martens A, et al. Partial tibial neurectomy in 113 Belgian blue calves with spastic paresis. Vet Rec 2000 Jul 1;147(1):16–9.
13. Weaver AD. Spastic paresis. In: Weaver AD, St Jean G, Steiner A, editors. Bovine surgery and lameness. 2nd edition. Oxford (UK): Blackwell; 2005. p. 246–8.
14. Greenough PR, Maccallum FJ, Weaver AD. Infectious diseases of deep structures. In: Greenough PR, Maccallum FJ, Weaver AD, editors. Lameness in cattle. Philadelphia: Lippincott; 1981. p. 176–96.
15. Greenough PR. Observations on some of the diseases of the bovine foot, Part II. Vet rec 1962;74:53–63.
16. Greenough PR, Maccallum FJ, Weaver AD. Diseases of muscles. In: Greenough PR, Maccallum FJ, Weaver AD, editors. Lameness in cattle. Philadelphia: Lippincott; 1981. p. 363–73.
17. Gillis C. Ultrasound diagnosis: tendon and ligament injury. Large Animal Vet 1993; July/August, 8–12.
18. Miles KG. Basic principles and clinical applications of diagnostic ultrasonography. Compend Contin Educ Pract Vet 1989;11:609–22.
19. Greenough PR, Maccallum FJ, Weaver AD. Diseases of horn and sensitive laminae. In: Greenough PR, Maccallum FJ, Weaver AD, editors. Lameness in cattle. Philadelphia: Lippincott; 1981. p. 170–96.
20. Homey FD, Amstutz HE. Musculoskeletal system. In: Amstutz HE, editor, Bovine medicine and surgery, vol. 2. Santa Barbara (CA): American Veterinary Publications; 1980. p. 863–85.
21. Johnson JH. The musculoskeletal system (muscles and tendons). In: Oehme FW, editor. Textbook of large animal surgery. 2nd edition. Baltimore (MD): Williams & Wilkins; 1988. p. 231–61.
22. Turner AS. Large animal orthopedics. In: Jennings PB, editor, The practice of large animal surgery, vol. II. Philadelphia: Saunders; 1984. p. 768–949.
23. Wheat JD, Asbury AC. Rupture of the gastrocnemius muscle in a cow—a case report. J Am Vet Med Assoc 1958;132:331–2.
24. Stashak TA. Lameness. In: Stashak TS, editor. Adam's lameness in horses. 4th edition. Philadelphia: Lea and Febiger; 1987. p. 764–7.
25. Wilson DC, Vanderby R. An evaluation of six synthetic casting materials: strength 01 cylinders in bending. Vet Surg 1995;24:55–9.
26. Wilson DC, Vanderby R. An evaluation of fiberglass application techniques. Vet Surg 1995;24:118–21.
27. Pasquini C. Thoracic limb. In: Pasquini C, editor. Atlas of bovine anatomy. Eureka (CA): Sudz Publishing; 1982. p. 203–43.
28. Pasquini C. Pelvic limb. In: Pasquini C, editor. Atlas of bovine anatomy. Eureka (CA): Sudz Publishing; 1982. p. 245–83.
29. Hago BED, Vaughan LC, Plummer JM, et al. Equine synovial tendon sheath and bursae: a transmission electron microscopic study. Equine Vet J 1991;23:4758.
30. Stanek C. Morphological, functional, chemical and clinical studies of diseases of the digital flexor tendon sheath in cattle. Wiener Tierarztliche Monatsschrift 1987; 74(12):397–412.

31. Van Pelt RW. Aseptic tenosynovitis in cattle. J Am Vet Med Assoc 1970;157:178–89.
32. Gaughan EM, Nixon AI, Krook LP, et al. Effects of sodium hyaluronate on tendon healing and adhesion formation in horses. Am J Vet Res 1991;52:764–73.
33. Barza M, Samuelson T, Weinstein L. Penetration of antibiotics into fibrin loci in vivo, II: comparison of nine antibiotics: effect of dose and degree of protein binding. J Infect Dis 1974;129:66–72.
34. Barza M, Weinstein L. Penetration of antibiotics into fibrin loci in vivo, I: comparison of penetration of ampicillin into fibrin clots, abscesses, and interstitial fluid. J Infect Dis 1974;129:59–65.
35. Hau T, Nishikawa RA, Phuangsab A. The effect of bacterial trapping by fibrin on the efficacy of systemic antibiotics in experimental peritonitis. Surg Gynecol Obstet 1983;157:252–6.
36. Baird AN, Scruggs OW, Watkins JP, et al. Effect of antimicrobial solution lavage on the palmar digital tendon sheath in horses. Am J Vet Res 1990;51:1488–94.
37. Bertone AL, McIlwraith CW, Powers BE, et al. Effect of four antimicrobial lavage solutions on the tarsocrural joint of horses. Vet Surg 1986;15:305–15.
38. Wilson DC, Cooley AJ, MacWilliams PS, et al. Effects of 0.05% chlorhexidine lavage on the tarsocrural *joints* of horses. Vet Surg 1994;23:442–7.
39. Smith JA, Williams RJ, Knight AP. Drug therapy for arthritis in food-producing animals. Compend Contin Educ Pract Vet 1989;11:87–94.
40. Walker RD, Richardson DC, Bryant MJ, et al. Anaerobic bacteria associated with osteomyelitis in domestic animals. J Am Vet Med Assoc 1983;182:814–6.
41. Bengtsson B, Franklin A, Luthman I, et al. Concentrations of sulphadimidine, oxytetracycline and penicillin G in serum, synovial fluid and tissue cage fluid after parenteral administration to calves. J Vet Pharmacol Ther 1989;12:37–45.
42. Gagnon H, Ferguson JG, Papich MG, et al. Single-dose pharmacoklnetlcs of cephazolin in bovine synovial fluid after intravenous regional Injection. J Vet Pharmacol Ther 1994;17:31–7.

Management of Fractures in Field Settings

David E. Anderson, DVM, MS[a,*], Guy St. Jean, DMV, MS[b]

KEYWORDS

• Fracture • Splint • Cast • External • Skeletal fixation • Pin cast

Limb fractures are common in farm animals, are most commonly found in young stock, and often occur subsequent to trauma during dystocia or handling. The most common fractures in food animals, such as cattle, include those of the metacarpus and metatarsus (approximately 50%), tibia (approximately 12%), radius and ulna (approximately 7%), and humerus (<5%). Fractures of the femur and pelvis also occur, but are uncommon. Fractures of the phalanges are rare.[1] Fractures of the axial skeleton (mandible, vertebra, ribs, pelvis) are even less common. Food animals are excellent patients for treatment of orthopaedic injuries because they spend a majority of time lying down, have a tremendous potential for bone healing, are more resistant than other animals to contralateral limb breakdown and stress laminitis, and usually do not resist having orthopedic devices on their limbs. The decision to treat a fracture in a food animal is made by considering the cost of the treatment, the success rate of the treatment, the perceived or potential economic or genetic value of the animal, and the location and type of fracture. Most owners elect inexpensive treatment for fractures with a high success rate. Owners also often elect costly fracture treatment, even when the success rate is estimated to be poor, when cattle are perceived to have high economic or genetic potential.

EMERGENCY TREATMENT

Temporary stabilization of limb fractures may be performed before moving the animal or attempting to get the animal to stand (**Fig. 1**). As a general rule, fractures below the level of the midradius or midtibia may be temporarily stabilized with splints or casts. In our experience, field stabilization of fractures proximal to this level should not be attempted. These efforts often result in the creation of a "fulcrum effect" at the fracture site and result in increased soft tissue trauma, damage to neurovascular structures, or compounding of the fracture. Cattle with these fractures should be carefully loaded

[a] Department of Clinical Sciences, College of Veterinary Medicine, Kansas State University, 1800 Denison Avenue, Manhattan, KS 66506, USA
[b] Ross University School of Veterinary Medicine, P.O. Box 334, Basseterre, St. Kitts, West Indies
* Corresponding author.
E-mail address: danderso@vet.ksu.edu (D.E. Anderson).

Vet Clin Food Anim 24 (2008) 567–582
doi:10.1016/j.cvfa.2008.07.006 vetfood.theclinics.com
0749-0720/08/$ – see front matter © 2008 Elsevier Inc. All rights reserved.

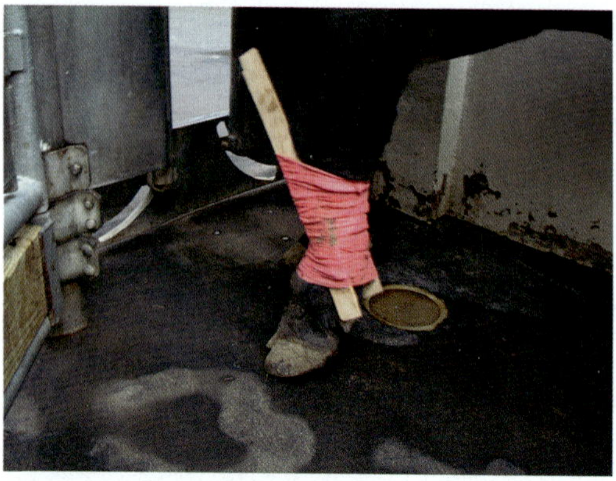

Fig. 1. Improper splint application for stabilization of a metacarpal fracture. Splint errors: Wooden splints are too small; splints are not placed 90° from each other; padding is inadequate; and insufficient bandaging tape is applied.

into a trailer and allowed to lie down before beginning transport. For these proximal injuries, cattle will protect the limb adequately for transport and any additional trauma that occurs is less severe than that which may occur as a result of the "fulcrum effect."

Two splints or a cast may be used to provide external coaptation for temporary stabilization of the fracture. Two boards or pieces of a large polyvinyl chloride (PVC) pipe cut in half and placed 90° to each other (eg, caudal and lateral aspect of the limb) create a stable external coaptation. A padded bandage is placed on the limb, the splints positioned, and elastic tape applied firmly. Circular clamps (eg, hose clamps) may be used to achieve firm placement of the splints on the limb. The injury should be centered within the coaptation with as much support proximal and distal to the injury as possible. All external coaptation devices should extend to the ground (to a level immediately distal to the sole of the hooves). For injuries distal to the carpus or hock, the splints should be placed to the level of the proximal radius or tibia, respectively. For injuries proximal to the carpus or hock and distal to the midradius or midtibia, the lateral splint should extend to the level of the proximal scapula or pelvis, respectively.

PRINCIPLES OF FRACTURE MANAGEMENT

The location of the fracture, presence or absence of soft tissue and neurovascular trauma, the status of the fracture environment (closed or open), the behavioral nature of the animal, and the experience of the veterinarian are important factors for considering what type of treatment is chosen. Fractures of the axial skeleton are often treated by stall rest alone because external or internal fixation is not required. For fractures involving the apendicular skeleton, the following questions must be answered: (1) Is treatment required? (2) Can the fracture be acceptably reduced closed or is internal reduction required? (3) Can the fracture be adequately immobilized using external coaptation alone, or is internal fixation, with or without external coaptation, required? And (4) What is the cost-benefit analysis?

Walking Block

Cattle have two weight-bearing digits for each limb. Therefore, a cow may stand on one digit during convalescence of the paired digit (eg, phalangeal fracture). A wooden, rubber, or plastic block (2.5 to 3.5 cm in height and formed to the size and shape of the healthy hoof) can be applied to the sole of the healthy digit (**Fig. 2**). A walking block is most suitable for management of P1, P2, and P3 fractures of a single digit. The animal is confined to a pen for 6 to 10 weeks while the fracture heals. If the block is present 6 weeks after placement, it should be removed. Often, wooden blocks become worn and removal is not necessary.

Casting

Half-limb casts (also called low-limb casts or short casts) can be used for immobilization of phalangeal fractures and for distal metacarpal or metatarsal physis fractures (**Fig. 3**). The cast is placed from a point immediately distal to the carpus or hock extending to the ground and encasing the foot. The dewclaws and the top of the cast are padded, but only stockinette or foam resin padding (eg, 3M Custom Support Foam, 3M Animal Care Products, St. Paul, Minnesota) is placed on the remainder of the limb. Thick padding, placed along the entire limb, quickly becomes compressed, leaving room for the limb to move within the cast and displacement of the fracture to occur. Full-limb casts (also called high-limb casts or long casts) are used for fractures occurring at or proximal to the midmetacarpus or metatarsus, but distal to the midradius or midtibia. Full limb casts are placed similarly to half-limb casts, but the bony prominences of the accessory carpal bone, styloid process of the ulna, calcaneous, and medial and lateral maleolus of the tibia must be padded.

A rope restraint, sedation, or anesthesia can be used as needed to facilitate placement of the cast. An assistant should help to maintain alignment of the limb during application, being sure to check the position of the limb in craniocaudal and lateromedial planes. Tension on the limb during casting may be achieved by placing wires through holes drilled in the hoof wall and applying tension. The holes should be placed such that the hoof is positioned in a normal to slightly flexed position. The thickness of the cast is usually based on clinical judgment. Casts 6 to 8 layers thick may be adequate for calves weighing less than 150 kg, but adult cattle may require casts 12 to 16 layers thick. Casts used on the hind limbs must be made thicker because of stress concentration by the angulation of the hock. Incorporation of metal rods within the cast (two rods placed 90° to each other) can increase the strength of the cast, but such rods are only needed in the largest of patients. Newer fiberglass casting materials are more resistant to breaking and do not weaken when wet if sufficient cast material is used. A walking bar (a U-shaped bar placed under the hoof and

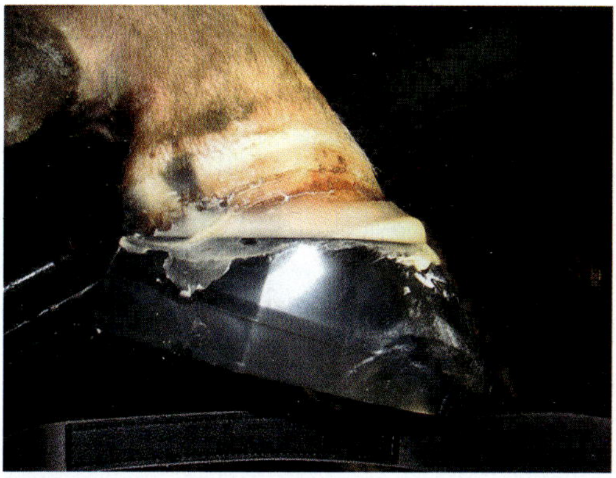

Fig. 2. Plastic walking block glued to sole surface and hoof wall of the healthy digit to allow limited weight-bearing on injured digit.

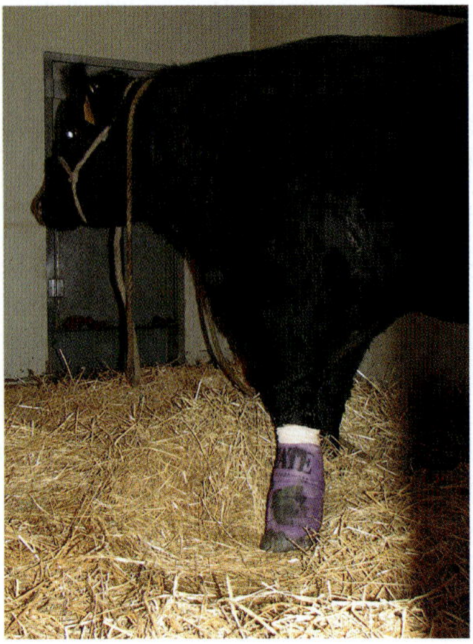

Fig. 3. Low-limb cast applied from the sole surface distally up to the midmetacarpus proximally for stabilization of a fracture of the second phalanx.

incorporated into the cast) concentrates loading forces into the cast and away from the distal limb, but the foot should always be included in the cast.

Casts may be maintained in calves for up to 6 weeks without being changed (**Fig. 4**). Scheduled cast changes at 3-week intervals may be required for rapidly growing calves or for calves that become lame during convalescence. Physeal fractures usually heal within 4 weeks, but nonphyseal fractures often require 6 weeks to reach clinical union in calves. Fractures in adult cattle may heal within 8 to 10 weeks, but often require 12 to 16 weeks for clinical union to occur. Radiographic union of the fracture (defined as bone union with resolution of the fracture line) is not seen for weeks to months after clinical union (defined as sufficient bridging callus to allow weight bearing without additional support to the limb) has been reached.

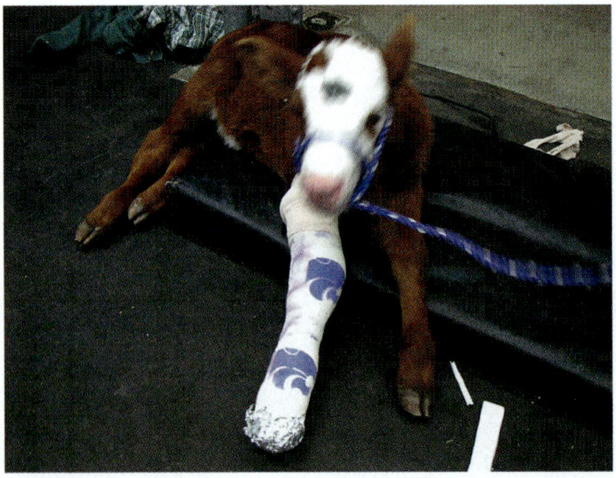

Fig. 4. Full-limb cast applied to a calf for stabilization of a fracture of the distal physis of the radius.

Thomas Splint and Cast Combination

Use of a Thomas splint and cast combination is appropriate for fractures distal to the elbow or stifle.[2] The length of the splint should be measured while the animal is standing and by using the normal limb for measurements. An appropriate splint is chosen or constructed, and the patient is placed into lateral recumbency (using rope restraint, sedation, anesthesia, or a combination of the three). The fracture is reduced and a cast applied from the distal metacarpus or metatarsus to the level of the proximal radius or tibia. The splint is placed on the limb, the foot is attached to the base of the splint by drilling holes in the hoof walls and wiring the foot to the splint base, and casting tape is used to attach the cast to the splint frame. The limb cast should be firmly attached to the splint frame to prevent rotation of the limb along the splint during ambulation. The hoop of the splint must be firmly placed into the axilla or groin to allow maximal weight transference. Therefore, the hoop must be heavily padded. Cattle having a Thomas splint-cast must be assisted to stand for 3 to 5 days until they learn how to rise under their own power (**Fig. 5**). Also, these patients must be checked several times daily to ensure that they have not lain down on top of the splint. Often patients are not able to rise after lying down on the splint and life-threatening rumen tympanities may occur if they remain trapped for a prolonged period.

Transfixation Pinning and Casting and External Skeletal Fixation

External skeletal fixation (ESF) refers to the stabilization of a debilitating musculoskeletal injury (typically fractures but also joint luxation or tendon rupture) using transfixation pins (or transcortical pins) and any external frame connecting the pins and spanning the region of instability.[3] The goal of transfixation pinning and casting (TPC) is to provide a sustainable, comfortable means to return the patient to weight bearing (or function) as soon as possible after surgery, to maintain normal joint mobility, if possible, and to provide an optimal environment for osteosynthesis and wound healing.

Mechanical breakdowns of external skeletal fixators include failure of the implants (bending or breaking of the pins), sidebars, or clamps because of acute failure or cyclical fatigue. These potential problems have contributed to the slow and cautious adaptation of ESF in large animals. Use of ESF in ruminants has also been impeded by

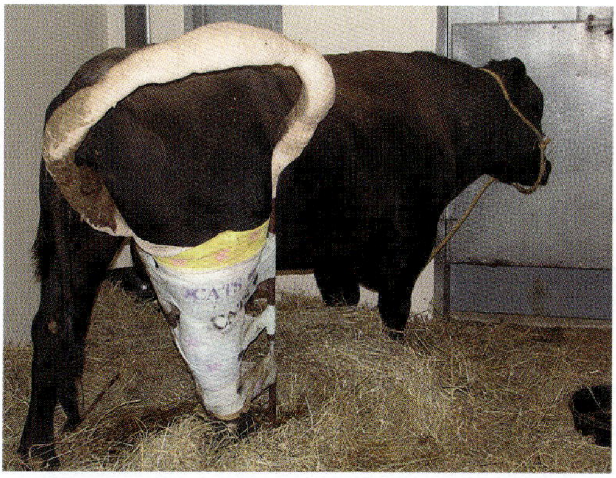

Fig. 5. Angus bull, age 2.5 years, weight 1000 kg, with a Thomas splint-cast combination used for stabilization of a Salter Harris type II fracture of the proximal tibia.

economic constraints. ESF is being increasingly used in cattle, sheep, goats, llamas, and ratites. This article explains how the principles of ESF are adapted to cattle, discusses the application of ESF to individual bones, and describes potential complications in the use of ESF.

DECISION-MAKING FOR EXTERNAL SKELETAL FIXATION

Cast immobilization often is appropriate for a fracture in an individual ruminant.[4] Complications of casting can include one or more of the following: muscle contracture; loss of range of motion of joints because of joint capsule and ligament contracture; reduction in articular cartilage quality and health because of prolonged immobilization; cast ulcers; impingement of soft tissues and vasculature; creation of open wounds that may communicate with the fracture; malalignment of the fracture; malunion of the fracture; delayed union of the fracture; and prolonged convalescence. With the proper use of ESF, these complications can be prevented or minimized. When cast immobilization is not appropriate or does not provide optimal management of fractures, other modalities must be considered. Casts cannot adequately immobilize fractures proximal to the distal radial physis or the distal tibial physis. Also, soft tissue injuries and open fractures may not be managed optimally by use of casts, splints, or splint-cast combinations. ESF presents a better option for stability and healing of fractures in many cases based on fracture configuration, soft tissue injuries, or open fractures. Usually, ESF is used in purebred cattle, show cattle, or other cattle of high perceived economic value.

Advantages

ESF has many advantages for the treatment of fractures.[5–11] ESF provides early return to function of the affected limb; accommodates management of soft tissue wounds on the limb; permits local blood flow to the fracture site; preserves bone stimulatory proteins that exude into the fracture site at the time of initial injury; allows diverse designs for treating comminuted fractures; permits easy implant removal after clinical union of the fracture; and results in relatively few complications from the implants. ESF has been applied to most of the long bones of the domestic species. Transarticular application of external fixators has been used in the presence of severe soft tissue trauma or severe comminution of the proximal or distal end of the affected bone, and for arthrodesis or ankylosis of joints.[12,13] Transarticular use of external fixators must be done with consideration for the potential of inducing damage to the involved joint because of immobilization.[14–16]

Disadvantages

Disadvantages of ESF are suboptimal fracture reduction and poor anatomic alignment, absence of interfragmentary compression, less rigid stabilization of the affected bone compared with bone plates, increased postoperative management compared with bone plates or casting, pain associated with micromotion at the pin-bone interface, and potential failure of the implants before clinical union of the fracture.

Whenever possible, transcortical pins should be inserted between muscles and through facial planes. Pins placed through major muscle groups may result in pain and reduced use of the affected limb. In a femoral fracture study, dogs returned to normal, full function within 3.5 weeks after application of a bone plate compared with 7.5 weeks after application of a intramuscular pin and half Kirchner splint.[7] Also, minimal intervening soft tissue between the sidebar and bone is desirable so that the bone-sidebar distance can be optimized.

GUIDELINES FOR EXTERNAL SKELETAL FIXATION IN FOOD ANIMALS

Fractures of the metacarpus/metatarsus III/IV, radius, ulna, and tibia may be most easily repaired using ESF with the patient in dorsal recumbency and the limb suspended from an overhead frame. Lateral recumbency is done with careful attention to alignment in the sagittal planes. Fractures of the humerus and femur are approached with the animal in lateral recumbency. Excessive soft tissue swelling and inflammation is typical of fractures in large animals. If the surgeon has little experience with ESF in ruminants, we suggest placement of marker needles at the proposed site for placement of the transcortical pins. Then, radiograph images are obtained and the pin sites are chosen based on the relationship of the marker needles with the fracture, fissure lines, adjacent joints, and intact cortical bone. With experience in choosing placement of pins and thorough knowledge of the limb anatomy of cattle, this step can be omitted.

A l-cm incision is made through the skin at the chosen pin site. A hole is then drilled through the bone and another incision is made for the exit site of the pin (for bilateral transcortical pins). We use a low-speed, high-torque battery drill with variable speeds. Pins are implanted with the drill at low speed. Sterility must be maintained either by gas sterilization of the drill or by coverage of the drill with sterile draping material. During drilling, the drill bit should be continuously flushed with a sterile isotonic solution to help decrease thermal injury to the bone. Finally, the pin is implanted. Selection of drill bit and pin sizes should be done such that the pin is large enough to sustain full ambulatory weight-loading by the patient. A tissue protector, or pin guide, is beneficial to prevent excessive soft tissue trauma during drilling and implantation.

Transfixation Pinning and Casting

TPC has been used successfully in cattle for fractures of various bones.[17–20] This adaptation of ESF techniques has the distinct advantage of multiplanar fixation with the placement of transfixation pins limited only by anatomic structures and fracture configuration. Also, TPC allows minimal postoperative case management with a high degree of success. This advantage is particularly suited to food animals.

We exclusively use fiberglass casting tape for TPC (**Fig. 6**). We have found that inclusion of metal braces or walking bars is not necessary when using fiberglass casts. Recent biomechanical studies have shown differences with application techniques for fiberglass casts and potential benefits of placing a metal bar on the compression and tension sides of the limb.[21,22] Clinical judgment is the best guide for the thickness of the cast. We have seen two full-limb rear-limb casts fail after surgery. Both failed at the dorsal aspect of the hock. The first cast failed when an adult bull with a tibial fracture tried to stand before the cast had completely dried. The other cast broke because of insufficient cast material to withstand the forces imparted by an adult bull. Both casts were repaired, and both bulls made a complete recovery.

Pin position and fixator configuration cannot be adjusted after the cast has been applied when using TPC. Also, open wounds or open fractures are difficult to manage with TPC. Complications during TPC, such as creation of an open fracture or development of cast sores, are difficult to assess and some delay may be required to address these problems. We recommend using resin-impregnated foam (eg, 3M Custom Support Foam) on the limb before casting. This foam padding conforms to the limb, provides excellent protection of the limb, and allows the limb to remain dry under the cast because of its porous structure. We have observed a decrease in the severity of pin tract complications when the foam padding was used.

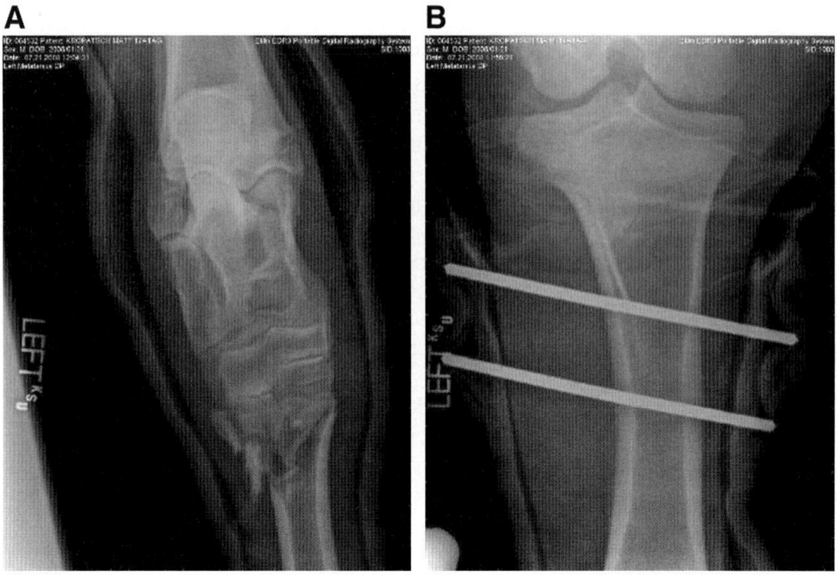

Fig. 6. (*A*) Comminuted, articular fracture of the proximal metacarpus III/IV in a 6-month-old bull calf. (*B*) Transfixation pin cast applied to stabilize fracture presented in *A*. Pins are placed through the mid- to proximal tibia and a full-limb cast applied incorporating the pins into the fiberglass casting tape.

Closed Versus Open Fractures

Overall, closed fractures without damage to the limb's blood supply have a good to excellent prognosis for healing in cattle. Open fractures have a guarded prognosis for healing in cattle. The success rate depends on the severity of soft tissue damage, the bone affected, the age of the patient, the duration and degree of contamination of the wound, and the economic limitations placed on fracture management. The prognosis for success is less in young calves, especially when significant damage is present, as often occurs with fractures caused by calving chains. Older cattle and heavy cattle have a more guarded prognosis because stabilization of the injury is more challenging. Prolonged antibiotic therapy is indicated, and open wound management is preferable to enclosing the wound within a cast. Compared to calves, mature cattle are better able to overcome bone infection associated with open fractures. Often, a mature cow with an open metacarpal fracture is able to heal and return to productivity after thorough cleaning of the wound, administration of antibiotics, and application of a full-limb cast. By contrast, a young calf with a similar injury is prone to septic nonunion or delayed union.

The management of open fractures presents special challenges to the surgeon. We consider all penetrating skin wounds associated with fractures to be infected because of the severity of contamination with dirt and manure typical of food animals. After induction of anesthesia, we clean and debride the wound, and copiously lavage the wound. Empiric antibiotic therapy is initiated at the time of surgery and continued until bacterial culture and sensitivity results are obtained. Antibiotic selection for use in cattle must be made with consideration for extralabel use and potential antibiotic residues.[23]

Empiric antibiotic therapy should be based on known osseous pathogens affecting cattle. The most common bacteria cultured from skeletal infections in cattle are

Arcanobacter pyogenes, Streptocccoccus spp, *Staphylococcus* spp, *Fusobacterium necrophorum, Bacteroides* spp, and coliforms.[24–29] Antibiotics proven to achieve therapeutic concentrations in bone include penicillin, cephalosporins, fluoroquinolones, and trimethoprim-sulfa combinations (age-dependent).[30–33] Based on our clinical experience and bacterial susceptibility results, we routinely initiate antibiotic therapy with procaine penicillin G (22,000 U/kg body weight, every 24 hours, subcutaneously or intramuscularly) or sodium ceftiofur (2.2 mg/kg body weight, every 24 hours, subcutaneous or intramuscular). At the time of this writing, extralabel use of cephalosporins in food animals was allowed under the Animal Medical Drug Use Clarification Act. However, the Food and Drug Administration announced in the summer of 2008 that extralabel use of cephalosporins would no longer be legal after October 1, 2008. As no antibiotics are labeled for use in bone infection in cattle, the options are limited to drugs with legal extralabel application.

When open wounds are present and adequate drainage established from the wound, we perform copious lavage frequently, depending on the degree of contamination and the severity of the infection. The wound, limb, and ESF are wrapped with clean bandage materials to prevent contamination from the environment. Sterile gauze padding is applied to the wound. We frequently use topical antiseptic ointments to cover the external wound. We feel that the potential benefit of topical antiseptics in preventing ascending infection outweighs mild inhibitory effects on wound healing. Daily wound care is continued until granulation tissue has covered the wound.

Chronic infection (osteomyelitis) of the fracture can be more difficult to resolve. Intravenous infusion of antibiotics distal to a tourniquet achieves high levels of antibiotics in synovial fluid and we have adapted this technique to the treatment of chronic osseous infections. Fractures caused by calving chain injuries and those having extensive soft tissue damage often are associated with osseous sequestra. Fracture healing is slowed by the presence of the sequestrum, and sequestrectomy usually allows fracture healing to procede. Definition of the sequestrum often is not apparent until 4 to 6 weeks after the initial injury. In calves having fracture of the metacarpus or metatarsus caused by injudicious use of calving chains, full cortical sequestra can be seen and often lead to nonunion or extreme delayed union. In these calves, we remove the sequestrum at the earliest time possible based on radiographs or clinical findings, cleanse the wound until a healthy granulation bed is present, and then perform cancellous bone grafting from the sternum. The sternum provides the largest volume of cancellous bone for grafting. Alternatively, the proximal tibia, proximal humerus, or ileum may be used for cancellous grafts.

Infected fractures that progress to septic nonunion should be treated similarly to cortical sequestrum cases. Aerobic and anaerobic cultures and microbial susceptibility tests aid in antibiotic selection and the fracture site is extensively debrided of fibrous tissue. The debridement is continued until healthy bone is exposed. A fresh, autologous cancellous bone graft is then harvested and implanted into the fracture site. We use a 4.5- to 6.0-mm drill bit to gain access to the medullary cavity of the normal bone. In cattle having chronic nonhealing fractures, failure to ambulate and altered weight bearing caused by lameness causes medullary atrophy. This limits the volume of cancellous bone that can be harvested from the long bones. Thus, we use the sternum as the site of choice for cancellous bone harvest if the procedure is to be performed under general anesthesia or using methods that prevent accidental trauma to the sternum or thorax. A bone curette is used to collect the maximum quantity of cancellous bone accessible. This bone is packed into the fracture and, if possible, the skin is closed over the site. This treatment is based on a similar technique used successfully to treat septic nonunion in humans.[34]

When the infection is too extensive for routine debridement and cancellous bone grafting or when the wound does not have a healthy granulation bed to provide blood supply to the graft, we perform extensive debridement and implant handmade antibiotic-impregnated beads. We prepare orthopedic-grade polymethylmethacrylate bone cement and then mix in powdered penicillin, sodium ceftiofur, cefazolin, or ampicillin before implanting the cement. Therapeutic concentrations may be achieved locally for more than 21 days after implantation.[35–39]

Septic nonunion may be successfully treated by rigid immobilization and the surgical techniques described above. However, the economic limitations of an individual animal may be encountered before clinical union of the fracture has occurred. Clinical union in these cases may require 6 to 8 months after injury.

Clinical Perspectives on Fractures Suitable for Treatment in Field Settings

Radius and ulna

Closed fractures of the distal physis of the radius may be treated by a full-limb cast and has a good prognosis for success. Fracture of the midradius and ulna requires use of a Thomas splint-cast, transfixation pin-cast, or bone plate. The prognosis for healing is good, but significant contralateral limb injury may occur in animals treated by the Thomas splint-cast. TPC and bone plating have good to excellent prognoses with minimal risk of permanent injury to the contralateral limb. Where applicable and economical, we prefer to treat fractures of the radius and ulna using TPC (**Fig. 7**).

The radius is well suited to ESF using TPC when the fracture is closed.[40–43] When fracture configuration allows placement of multiple pins proximal and distal to the fracture and the patient weighs less than 150 kg, we place the cast spanning the antebrachium only. This allows free movement of all joints in the forelimb. In patients weighing more than 150 kg, we use a full-limb cast to provide additional support to the assembly. When the fracture is open, we use ESF with metal or acrylic sidebars to provide access to the wound for daily fracture management. Septic osteomyelitis may lead to destruction of the patient if extensive debridement and wound care are not performed.

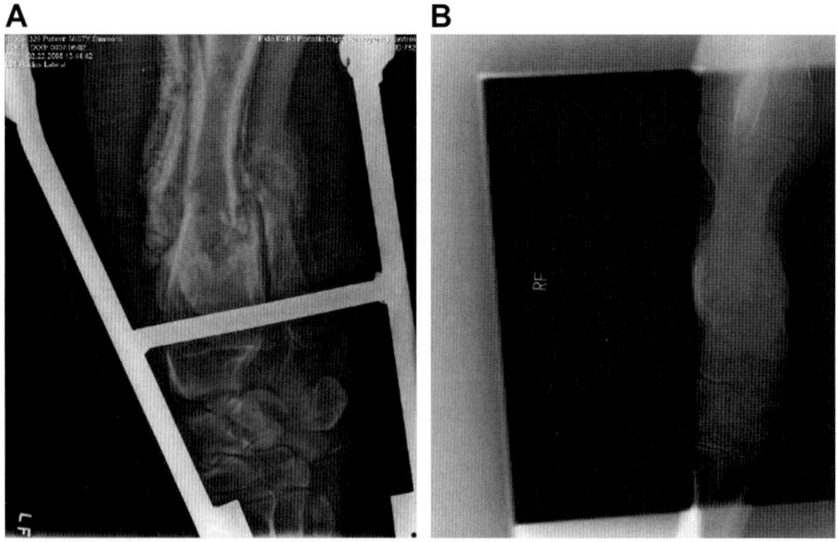

Fig. 7. (*A*) Thomas splint-cast used to stabilize a distal radius/ulna fracture in a calf. (*B*) Clinical union of radius/ulna fracture 8 weeks after application of a Thomas splint-cast combination.

In the authors' experience, most open radial fractures involve the distal diaphysis or physis. A type II, transarticular ESF is necessary to stabilize the fracture because of the small size and irregular geometry of the distal radial epiphysis. Two or three pins are placed into the diaphysis of the proximal radius, one pin may be placed into the distal radial epiphysis, and two or three pins are placed into the diaphysis of the metacarpus III/IV. The ESF should be maintained until the infection has resolved and clinical bone union is achieved. Clinical union is expected within 4 to 6 weeks in calves and within 8 to 10 weeks in adults after stabilization. Open fractures may require 12 weeks or more for clinical bone union. Clinical bone union refers to fracture stability sufficient to allow ambulation without external support, but with incomplete osseous remodeling.

Placement of transcortical pins through the radius should be done in the fascial plane between the lateral digital extensor muscle and the ulnaris lateralis muscle (placement from lateral to medial direction). The principle neurovascular structures of the antebrachium are located on the caudomedial aspect of the radius. Therefore, placement of pins through the center of the radius in a lateral-to-medial direction has minimal risk of damaging these vessels and nerves. Multiplanar unilateral pins may be placed into the radius with the aid of palpation, marker pins, and intraoperative radiographs to estimate the optimal position for the pins. When casting is not used, the sidebars are placed so that a 1-cm space exists between the skin and sidebar at the closest point (usually the distal radial metaphysis).

Tibia

Although fracture of the tibia has been seen as a result of forced extraction during dystocia, tibia fractures are usually caused by trauma. Fracture of the distal physis of the tibia may be treated with a full-limb cast, but these fractures are uncommon. Fracture of the middle portion of the tibia may be treated by a Thomas splint-cast, TPC, or use of a bone plate.[1–3] Thomas splint-casts have a good prognosis for bone healing, but have a high rate of injury to the contralateral limb. Transfixation pin-casts and bone plates have a good to excellent prognosis for healing, and pose minimal problems with contralateral limb injury.

Fracture of the tibia is the most common fracture treated by TPC in cattle. Use of a modified Thomas splint-cast combination is associated with multiple short-term and long-term complications.[3] TPC of tibial fractures can be successful in cattle and we have used this in cattle weighing up to 1000 kg (2200 lb).[44–47]

Transfixation pins are more difficult to place correctly in the tibia compared with the metacarpus or metatarsus because of the extensive soft tissue coverage of the cranial, lateral, and caudal aspects of the bone. The principal neurovascular structures of the pelvic limb are located on the caudomedial aspect of the tibia. Therefore, lateral-to-medial transfixation pins may be placed with minimal risk of neurovascular trauma. Ideally, transfixation pins should be implanted, from lateral to medial, between the muscles and through fascial planes to minimize postoperative pain associated with muscle interference. However, the fascial planes between muscles surrounding the tibia are difficult to palpate and extensive swelling associated with inflammation and fracture hematoma makes palpation of these structures difficult. Therefore, we place transfixation pins based primarily on the fracture configuration with accommodation to soft tissues made when possible.

In calves weighing less than 150 kg, TPC may be place solely on the injured bone to optimize joint mobility. Two to three pins are placed proximal and distal to the fracture and fiberglass cast material is applied to span the length of the tibia. We usually cut a segment out of the caudal portion of the cast to allow free movement of the calcaneal tendons. Normal ambulation is afforded by this technique. Cattle weighing more than

150 kg require construction of a full-limb cast in support of the transfixing pins to optimize fracture stability.

Metacarpus and metatarsus III/IV

Fractures involving the metacarpus or metatarsus III/IV are the most common fractures in food animals. These injuries often occur as a result of forced extraction during dystocia. Closed fracture of the distal physis of the metacarpus or metatarsus may be treated using a half-limb cast. Closed fracture of the middle portion of the metacarpus or metatarsus may be treated with a full-limb cast. Open fractures in mature cattle may be treated by thoroughly debriding, cleaning, and flushing the wound, applying a full-limb cast, and administering antibiotics for 10 to 14 days. In valuable cattle and young calves, open fractures are best treated by use of an external skeletal fixator and daily wound care until the wound is healed. Bone sequestra are often associated with open fractures of the metacarpus and metatarsus. Bone healing may not occur until sequestra have been removed. If prolonged sepsis has been present, cancellous bone grafts may be required to facilitate bone union. The optimal site for harvesting cancellous bone grafts are the wing of the ileum and the proximal tibia. Implantation of antibiotic-impregnated bone cement beads into a septic wound provides prolonged local release of antibiotics and may accelerate resolution of osteomyelitis.

The large metacarpal and metatarsal bones are readily suited for ESF because these bones have minimal soft tissue covering and the principle neurovascular tissues are located caudolateral and caudomedial to the bones. Therefore, transfixation pin placement is easily chosen without the aid of radiographs. We use radiographs only to determine the location of the fracture fragments and fissure lines relative to the pins. Most fractures of the metacarpus/metatarsus III/IV respond favorably to external coaptation. ESF is indicated for treatment of open, infected fractures or highly comminuted, inherently unstable fractures in cattle of high economic value. We often use TPC for closed fractures when the configuration of the fracture causes inherent instability or cosmetic concerns make casting less desirable. With TPC, the cast may be placed to span only the metacarpal/metatarsal region if (1) the patient weighs less than 150 kg and (2) there is sufficient bone proximal to the fracture to allow at least two suitably sized transfixing pins. This allows optimal ambulation. A full-limb TPC cast should be used in heavier patients to increase the stability of the assembly.

The prognosis for closed metacarpus/metatarsus III/IV fractures is fair to excellent with TPC. Animals treated with a walking cast (transfixation pins plus a metal frame within the cast) have good long-term productivity.[48,49] Use of TPC improves the prognosis for healing of open fractures, as compared with casting or Thomas splints, because of superior stability of the fracture site.

Complications of Casting and Splinting of Fractures

The most common complications of fracture are sepsis, nerve injury, and vascular injury. The most common complications of fracture treatment are cast or splint sores, breakdown injury in the contralateral limb, and malunion. Septic nonunion may occur from a combination of factors involved with fracture and fracture treatment. Nerve and vascular injury can be minimized by appropriate fracture immobilization before transporting the animal for definitive fracture treatment. Sepsis can be minimized by close attention to detail, thorough cleaning of the fracture site, and selection of appropriate antimicrobial drugs. Microbial cultures should be performed on all open fractures where economic limitations are not severe. Bone cultures are preferred to wound cultures for selection of antimicrobial drugs. Malunion can be prevented by optimal closed reduction or by open reduction and internal fixation when closed reduction cannot be achieved. Contralateral limb injury can be prevented by strict confinement of the animal during convalescence, frequent monitoring, removal of external coaptation at the earliest appropriate time, and client education for on-farm fracture-patient management.

COMPLICATIONS ASSOCIATED WITH EXTERNAL SKELETAL FIXATION

The most common clinical complications associated with ESF are instability at the fracture site, pin loosening, pin tract osteolysis, pin tract infections, implant failure, osteomyelitis, and delayed union or nonunion of the fracture.[50–55] ESF in ruminants has most commonly been performed using cast material as the external supporting frame for the pins (TPC).[17,33,41,44,52,56–59] The most common complications were pin tract osteolysis, pin loosening, and pin tract sepsis. In our experience in cattle, more than 50% of pins used in ESF become loose within 6 to 8 weeks. Pin site pain associated with loosening occurs in cattle, but pin pain does not often result in clinically significant problems in cattle as compared with horses. Cattle rest in sternal recumbency during most of the time of fracture convalescence. This repose markedly lessens pain associated with weight bearing and thus allows prolongation of the useful lifetime of ESF. Although common, pin tract osteolysis and pin tract infection rarely present a problem for resolution of the fracture. At the time of clinical union, pins are removed and the pin tracts are cleansed. Antibiotics may or may not be indicated. Pin tracts heal rapidly with little aftercare.

We have observed fractures of the radius in several cattle in which transfixation pins were used. These fractures invariably occur in the radius through the distal pin holes and may occur during ESF or after a TPC had been removed. Previously, we used full-limb casts after removal of the ESF in an attempt to protect the radius from being loaded in such a way that a pin hole fracture may occur. However, this type of staged removal of the external coaptation has not significantly lessened the likelihood of radius pin-hole fracture in our experience. The cast may serve as a fulcrum in which excessive focal loading of the pin hole can occur.

REFERENCES

1. Ferguson JG. Management and repair of bovine fractures. Compendium on Continuing Education for Practicing Veterinarians 1982;4:S128–35.
2. Anderson DE, St-Jean G. External skeletal fixation in ruminants. Vet Clin North Am Food Anim Pract 1996;12:117–52.
3. Anderson DE, St-Jean G, Vestweber JG, et al. Use of a Thomas splint-cast combination for stabilization of tibial fractures in cattle: 21 cases (1973–1993). Agri-Practice 1994;15:16–23.
4. Denny HR, Sridhar B, Weaver BM, et al. The management of bovine fractures: a review of 59 cases. Vet Rec 1988;123:289–95.
5. Aron DN, Toombs JP. Updated principles of external skeletal fixation. Compendium on Continuing Education for Practicing Veterinarians 1984;6:845–58.
6. Behrens F, Searls K. External fixation of the tibia. J Bone Joint Surg 1986;68B:246–54.
7. Braden TD, Brinker WO. Effect of internal fixation devices on functional limb usage in dogs. J Am Vet Med Assoc 1973;162:642–6.
8. Braden TD, Brinker WO, Little RW, et al. Comparative biomechanical evaluation of bone healing in the dog. J Am Vet Med Assoc 1973;163:65–9.
9. Nunamaker OM, Richardson OW, Butterweck OM, et al. A new external skeletal fixation device that allows immediate full weightbearing application in the horse. Vet Surg 1986;15:345–55.

10. Palmer RH, Hulse OA, Hyman WA, et al. Principles of bone haling and biomechanics of external skeletal fixation. Vet Clin North Am Small Anim Pract 1992; 22:45–8.
11. Richardson OW, Nunamaker OM, Sigafoos RO. Use of an external skeletal fixation device and bone graft for arthrodesis of the metacarpophalangeal joint in horses. J Am Vet Med Assoc 1987;191:316–21.
12. Bjorling DE, Toombs JP. Transarticular application of the Kirschner-Ehmer splint. Vet Surg 1982;11:34–8.
13. Toombs JP. Transarticular application of external skeletal fixation. Vet Clin North Am Small Anim Pract 1992;22:181–94.
14. Akeson WH, Amiel D, Abel MF, et al. Effects of immobilization on joints. Clin Orthop Relat Res 1987;219:28–37.
15. Kiviranta I, Tammi M, Jurbelin J, et al. Articular cartilage thickness and glycosaminogiycan distribution in the young canine knee joint after remobilization of the immobilized limb. J Orthop Res 1994;12:161–7.
16. Videman T, Michelsson JE, Rauhamaki R, et al. Changes in 35S-sulfate uptake in different tissues in the knee and hip regions of rabbits during immobilization, remobilization and the development of osteoarthritis. Acta Orthop Scand 1976; 47:290–8.
17. Kaneps AJ, Schmotzer WB, Huber MJ, et al. Fracture repair with transfixation pins and fiberglass cast in llamas and small ruminants. J Am Vet Med Assoc 1989; 195:1257–61.
18. Lundvall RL. Fractures of the long bones in large animals. J Am Vet Med Assoc 1960;137:308–12.
19. Reichel EC. Treatment of fractures of the long bones in large animals. J Am Vet Med Assoc 1956;103:8–15.
20. Saint-Jean G, Saint-Pierre H, Lamothe P, et al. Fractures epiphysaires et des os longs chez les ruminants. Medice Veterinaire Quebec 1985;15:63–77.
21. Wilson DC, Vanderby R. An evaluation of six synthetic casting materials: strength 01 cylinders in bending. Vet Surg 1995;24:55–9.
22. Wilson DC, Vanderby R. An evaluation of fiberglass application techniques. Vet Surg 1995;24:118–21.
23. Riviere JE. Practical aspects of the pharmacology of antimicrobial drug residues in food animals. Agri-Practice 1992;13:11–6.
24. Baird JD. Surgical treatment of osteomyelitis in a heifer. Aust Vet J 1973;49:202–4.
25. Merkens HW, van Dieten JSMM, Kerjes AW. Infectious (septic) arthritis of the distal interphalangeal and tarsometatarsal joint in cattle. Vet Rec 1984;114:212–3.
26. Rudman J, Fessler JF, Blevins WE, et al. Hematogenous osteomyelitis caused by *Fusobacterium neerophorum* in a calf. J Am Vet Med Assoc 1982;180:944–7.
27. Smith JA, Williams RJ, Knight AP. Drug therapy for arthritis in food-producing animals. Compendium on Continuing Education for Practicing Veterinarians 1989;11:87–94.
28. van de Watering Cc, Morgan JP, Kersjes AW. Radiographic diagnosis of *Corynebacterium pyogenes* bone infection in cattle. J Am Vet Radiol Soc 1976;2751–6.
29. Walker RD, Richardson DC, Bryant MJ, et al. Anaerobic bacteria associated with osteomyelitis in domestic animals. J Am Vet Med Assoc 1983;182:814–6.
30. Budsburg Sc, Kemp DT. Antimicrobial distribution and therapeutics in bone. Compendium on Continuing Education for Practicing Veterinarians 1990;12: 1758–63.
31. Duval JM, Budsberg SC. Cortical bone concentrations of emofloxacin in dogs. Am J Vet Res 1995;56:188–92.

32. Guard CL, Schwark WS, Friedman DS, et al. Age-related alterations in trimethoprimsulfadiazine disposition following oral or parenteral administration in calves. Can J Vet Res 1986;50:342–6.
33. Hanie EA. Antibiotic therapy for infections of skeletal and synovial structures, part II. Equine Practice 1989;11:7–14.
34. Green SA, Dlabal TA. The open bone graft for septic nonunion. Clin Orthop Relat Res 1983;180:117–24.
35. Adams K, Couch L, Cierny G, et al. In vitro and in vivo evaluation of antibiotic diffusion from antibiotic-impregnated polymethylmethacrylate beads. Clin Orthop Relat Res 1992;278:244–52.
36. Baker AS, Greenham LW. Release of gentamicin from acrylic bone cement. J Bone Joint Surg 1988;70A:1551–7.
37. DiMaio FR, O'Halloran JJ, Quale JM. In vitro elution of ciprofloxacin from polymethylmethacrylate cement beads. J Orthop Res 1994;12:79–82.
38. Miclau T, Oahners LE, Lindsey RW. In vitro pharmacokinetics of antibiotic release from locally implantable materials. J Orthop Res 1993;11:627–32.
39. Seligson O, Popham GJ, Voos K, et al. Antibiotic-leaching from polymethylmethacrylate beads. J Bone Joint Surg 1993;75A:714–9.
40. Anderson DE, St-Jean G, Desrochers A. Repair of open, comminuted fractures of the radius and ulna in a calf with a transarticular type II external skeletal fixator. AgriPractice 1994;15:24–8.
41. Baxter GM, Wallace CE. Modified transfixation pinning of compound radius and ulna fracture in a heifer. J Am Vet Med Assoc 1991;198:665–8.
42. St-Jean G, DeBowes RM. Transfixation pinning and casting of radial-ulnar fractures in calves: a review of three cases. Can Vet J 1992;33:257–62.
43. Hamilton GF, Tulleners EP. Transfixation pinning of proximal tibial fractures in calves. J Am Vet Med Assoc 1980;176:725–7.
44. St-Jean G, Clem MF, OeBowes RM. Transfixation pinning and casting of tibial fractures in calves: five cases (1985–1989). J Am Vet Med Assoc 1991;198: 139–43.
45. Verschooten F, De Moor A, Desmet P, et al. Surgical treatment of tibial fractures in cattle. Vet Rec 1972;90:24–9.
46. Vijaykumar OS, Singh AP, Nigam JM, et al. Repair of bovine tibial fractures. Vet Med Small Anim Clin 1982;77:1109–14.
47. Steiner A, Iselin U, Auer JA, et al. Shaft fractures of the metacarpus and metatarsus in cattle. Vet Comp Orthop Traumatol 1993;6:138–45.
48. Steiner A, Iselin U, Auer JA, et al. Physeal fractures of the metacarpus and metatarsus in cattle. Vet Comp Orthop Traumatol 1993;6:131–7.
49. Aron DN, Toombs IP, Hollingsworth SC. Primary treatment of severe fractures by external skeletal fixation: threaded pins compared with smooth pins. J Am Anim Hosp Assoc 1986;22:659–70.
50. Green SA, Ripley MJ. Chronic osteomyelitis in pin tracks. J Bone Joint Surg 1984; 66A:1092–8.
51. Johnson AL, Kneller SK, Weigel RM. Radial and tibial fracture repair with external skeletal fixation: effects of fracture type, reduction, and complications on healing. Vet Surg 1989;18:367–72.
52. Maurer OJ, Merkow RL, Gustilo RB. Infection after intramedullary nailing of severe open tibial fractures initially treated with external fixation. J Bone Joint Surg 1989; 71A:835–8.
53. Palmer RH, Aron DN. Ellis pin complications in seven dogs. Vet Surg 1990;19: 440–4.

54. Hench LL, Wilson J. Surface-active biomaterials. Science 1984;226:630.
55. Holmberg DL. The use of prophylactic penicillin in orthopedic surgery: a clinical trial. Vet Surg 1985;14:160–5.
56. Hoffsis GF, Henry SC. Extralabel use of veterinary drugs. Compendium on Continuing Education for Practicing Veterinarians 1988;10:1215–22.
57. Hyldahl C, Pearson S, Tepic S, et al. Induction and prevention of pin loosening in external fixators in the sheep tibia. In Proceedings of 34th Annual Meeting of the Orthopaedic Research Society, 1988. p. 304.
58. Ilizarov GA. Clinical application of the tension-stress effect for limb lengthening. Clin Orthop Relat Res 1990;250:8–25.
59. Johnson WD, Fischer DA. Skeletal stabilization with a multiplane external fixation device: biomechanical evaluation and finite element model. Clin Orthop Relat Res 1983;180:34–43.

Index

Note: Page numbers of article titles are in **boldface** type.

Vet Clin Food Anim 24 (2008) 583–593
doi:10.1016/S0749-0720(08)00073-X vetfood.theclinics.com
0749-0720/08/$ – see front matter © 2008 Elsevier Inc. All rights reserved.

D

E

P

R

T

V

W

X